P9-CFQ-298

Praise for *Sprout Right*

"Once you put down your pregnancy test, you should pick up *Sprout Right* ... this is a must read."

> —Alyson Schafer, parenting expert and author of *Honey, I Wrecked the Kids*

"Expectant moms and new parents are bombarded with nutrition information from so many different sources—it's tough to know whether we're doing the right thing. Lianne's voice stands out amid the din for its calm, informed and friendly assurance."

> —Sandra E. Martin, Senior Editor, *Today's Parent*

"Lianne Phillipson-Webb has written a comprehensive and mom-friendly guide to prenatal, infant, and toddler nutrition. The nutrient-packed recipes will be much appreciated by time-pressed but health-conscious moms."

> —Ann Douglas, author of *The Mother of All Pregnancy Books*

"Lianne offers valuable options and resources as well as amazing recipes that any child will enjoy."

> —Tracey Ruiz, CLD, CPD, CCCE

"The perfect, complete and reliable nutrition reference—this book is a blessing for any expecting woman or new mom."

> —Dr. Natasha Turner, ND, bestselling author of *The Hormone Diet*

"How I wish *Sprout Right: Nutrition from Tummy to Toddler* was around when my three children were babies. It's a fantastic resource about nutrition for expecting and new moms—the only book you'll need in your kitchen."

> —Sarah Morgenstern, publisher and co-founder, SavvyMom.ca

PENGUIN CANADA

SPROUT RIGHT

LIANNE PHILLIPSON-WEBB is the founder of Sprout Right, a company that specializes in pre-conception, prenatal, and postnatal nutrition for women, as well as good food and health for the whole family. With over ten years of experience, Lianne is a registered nutritionist, member of the International Organization of Nutrition Consultants, and mother of two.

Lianne graduated with honours from the Institute of Optimum Nutrition in London, England, and has since shared her knowledge with thousands of women and their families through personal consultations and numerous television appearances on *Canada AM, Breakfast Television,* Rogers, and *CHCH Morning Live.* She also contributes to *Today's Parent* magazine and many online parenting websites, runs Sprout Right's interactive workshops and one-of-a-kind Mommy Chef cooking classes, and produced an instructional DVD series.

Lianne is passionate about the environment. Her commitment to a healthy, environmentally balanced lifestyle is reflected in both her personal life and the Sprout Right philosophy. Organic food, recycling, and environmental conservation are all integrated into the workshops and cooking classes.

Lianne has a number of interests outside of nutrition. She is the mother of two daughters, and an active contributor to their school programs, as well as an IFR reflexologist, aromatherapist, and Reiki master.

Sprout Right

Nutrition from
Tummy to Toddler

Lianne Phillipson-Webb
REGISTERED NUTRITIONIST

PENGUIN
CANADA

PENGUIN CANADA

Published by the Penguin Group

Penguin Group (Canada), 90 Eglinton Avenue East, Suite 700, Toronto, Ontario, Canada
M4P 2Y3 (a division of Pearson Canada Inc.)

Penguin Group (USA) Inc., 375 Hudson Street, New York, New York 10014, U.S.A.
Penguin Books Ltd, 80 Strand, London WC2R 0RL, England
Penguin Ireland, 25 St Stephen's Green, Dublin 2, Ireland (a division of Penguin Books Ltd)
Penguin Group (Australia), 250 Camberwell Road, Camberwell, Victoria 3124, Australia
(a division of Pearson Australia Group Pty Ltd)
Penguin Books India Pvt Ltd, 11 Community Centre, Panchsheel Park, New Delhi – 110 017, India
Penguin Group (NZ), 67 Apollo Drive, Rosedale, North Shore 0745, Auckland, New Zealand
(a division of Pearson New Zealand Ltd)
Penguin Books (South Africa) (Pty) Ltd, 24 Sturdee Avenue, Rosebank, Johannesburg 2196,
South Africa

Penguin Books Ltd, Registered Offices: 80 Strand, London WC2R 0RL, England

First published 2010

2 3 4 5 6 7 8 9 10 (CR)

Copyright © Lianne Phillipson-Webb, 2010

Sprout Right™ and Mommy Chef™ are registered trademarks of Lianne Phillipson-Webb
and are used under licence.

All rights reserved. Without limiting the rights under copyright reserved above, no part of this
publication may be reproduced, stored in or introduced into a retrieval system, or transmitted
in any form or by any means (electronic, mechanical, photocopying, recording or otherwise),
without the prior written permission of both the copyright owner and the above publisher of
this book.

Manufactured in the U.S.A.

LIBRARY AND ARCHIVES CANADA CATALOGUING IN PUBLICATION

Phillipson-Webb, Lianne
Sprout right : nutrition from tummy to toddler / Lianne Phillipson-Webb.

Includes index.
ISBN 978-0-14-317350-2

1. Infants—Nutrition. 2. Toddlers--Nutrition. 3. Infants—
Health and hygiene. 4. Toddlers—Health and hygiene. 5. Cookery
(Baby foods). I. Title.

RJ206.P53 2010   613.2083   C2010-901153-8

Visit the Penguin Group (Canada) website at **www.penguin.ca**

Special and corporate bulk purchase rates available; please see **www.penguin.ca/corporatesales** or
call 1-800-810-3104, ext. 2477 or 2474

For my daughters, Logan and Hadley—you are my inspiration.

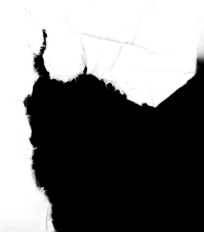

CONTENTS

INTRODUCTION

Congratulations on entering this new stage of your life—parenthood. I applaud you for your interest in learning about what great nutrition is and why it's important for your new family or family-to-be.

I'm passionate about good food but also about helping you understand why it's important to feed you and your baby well. If you don't know the nutritional benefits of leafy green vegetables, why would you put them on the menu? A good diet is synergistic with good health, and since you eat at least three times a day (ideally more), it's important to make what you eat count.

You'll find in this book many new concepts, suggestions, and ingredients, combined with super-nutritious, great-tasting recipes for your family. My goal is to motivate and guide you to an easy, healthy way to feed your baby or toddler. But first, I'll paint a picture of what's really going on inside your child's little body. For instance, what's her immune system up to, and how does it work? If it's not in tip-top shape, what are the implications? And most importantly, how can you support it nutritionally to function at its best? Everything written in this book has come from years of experience and research, not only as a nutritionist, but also as a mom of two amazing daughters.

In my work, I've taught many new parents who are eager to learn everything they can about the best way to feed their babies and toddlers and have somehow ended up in one of my cooking classes or workshops, or at my desk for a consultation. Even if they've come in to learn how to make baby food, I see and hear about positive changes in the rest of the family's diet (beginning with the parents!) as they become more aware of what good nutrition is and become better eaters themselves.

My daughters are my inspiration as well as my best critics. They've eaten every recipe in this book and given their own feedback by spitting it out, throwing it off the high chair, or gobbling it up; using sign language to ask for more (before they could talk); or, now, saying, "Wow, Mommy, your recipes are the best!"

In this book, I'll dig deep into crucial nutritional topics such as breastfeeding and formula-feeding, the immune system, the digestive system (as well as the end result: what you see in the diaper), and, of course, feeding your child. Other areas of the book are more instructional, with step-by-step suggestions for feeding mom and baby, as well as tried and tested recipes for nutritious baby and toddler food from my Mommy Chef cooking classes.

I hope you'll find the information in this book useful, as so many of my workshop attendees, Mommy Chefs, and private clients have over the past five years. I'm always so impressed with how the moms in my classes take on new ideas that are sometimes hard to wrap their heads around (probiotics, for instance), even while they're sleep deprived and busy entertaining their babies. And when a baby's eczema improves, a baby starts pooing without pain or screaming, or I hear back from a mom that her toddler is growing up healthy and strong because of what she learned in the Mommy Chef classes, I feel so proud that those parents have taken what they learned, implemented it, and seen for themselves how they can positively influence their children's health. And as you read this book, I hope you will too.

1

WHILE IN MOM'S TUM
Through Your Trimesters

Ideally, the reason you've picked up this book and are reading this first chapter hasn't come as a shock to you. If you've been planning a pregnancy, you've been getting your body into tip-top shape with pre-conceptual care, taking your vitamins (folic acid, especially), cutting out alcohol, and eating really well. But if your happy news has come as a surprise, don't worry—it's not too late to start planning for the healthiest pregnancy possible. Now that you've missed your period, the pregnancy test is positive, and you know the expected due date of your baby, it's time to celebrate. Congratulations!

You're about to embark on an exciting new stage of your life. Becoming a parent is amazing, mind-blowing, and worrying, all at the same time. You might feel at times that everyone has something to advise or share with you about being pregnant. It can be overwhelming trying to understand what's happening to your body and wondering how much of a difference what you drink, eat, and do over the next nine months will make to your developing baby. Well, there is increasing evidence that this stage of your baby's life (although still in your tum) may be the most important and influential one in helping to lessen the potential for disease later in life. Researchers are now saying that this is the time when "good health for life" actually starts. Don't worry about doing everything right—that's much too stressful. But the advice and suggestions in this chapter can help guide you on the right path to making great choices. You'll learn how to get the key nutrients you and baby need, understand why they're important, learn how to eat for two, and find out everything else you need to know have the healthiest pregnancy possible.

GETTING OFF TO A GOOD START: THE FIRST TRIMESTER

Immediately after the sperm and egg meet, thousands of cell divisions take place inside the womb (also known as the uterus). The first, very important developmental stage of the fetus is the formation of the brain, spinal cord, heart, and gastrointestinal tract. Amazingly, all of this will have happened before you've done your first pregnancy test. About halfway through your first 12 weeks, the lungs are forming, and the jaw and nose have begun to develop. At 8 weeks (6 weeks' gestation) your baby has everything your body does, including bones and muscles that contract. The baby continues to grow to about 3 centimetres by the time you're 12 weeks pregnant.

Working Out Your Due Date

Knowing when you ovulated or conceived might give you a more accurate due date. If you do know, count 266 days or 38 weeks forward to get that date. *Gestation* is a term used to describe the actual age of your baby, counting forward from conception, when sperm met the egg. Your doctor or midwife will ask the date of your last period, and then count forward by 40 weeks, which is the average duration of pregnancy. After your first ultrasound, between 11 and 13 weeks, that date might change to a more accurate one, based on the size of your baby.

This can be a very difficult time to concentrate on eating well, as you may be feeling sick. But whether you're nauseated or not, good nutrition is important in your first trimester. I've provided some guidelines to follow as best you can (depending on how you feel) to get a great start to your healthy pregnancy.

DEALING WITH "NOT ONLY IN THE MORNING" SICKNESS

The term *morning sickness* is—unfortunately—not tied to a particular time of day. Queasiness, nausea, and vomiting can happen at any time of day or, for some, all day long (I feel for you). Pregnancy sickness, as it's also sometimes called, can start at 4 weeks, but more commonly begins around 6 weeks and lasts until between 12 and 16 weeks. For some it lasts the duration of the pregnancy; others are lucky to avoid it altogether. If you're a lucky one, be thankful, and don't worry that it's a sign there might be something wrong. Everyone is different and has varying symptoms. Some say nausea is a good sign, although I'm sure that's not how you would describe it!

The cause of pregnancy sickness isn't completely understood, which is frustrating. One theory is that it's caused by the increase of a hormone called human chorionic gonadotropin, or hCG (the hormone that's present in urine about 12 to 14 days after conception and that makes your test show positive). The level of hCG in your blood increases as the baby develops. This hormone is produced by the developing placenta, which provides all of your baby's nutrition, including iron, zinc, calcium, vitamin D, and DHA, for the next nine months or so. Your body becomes flooded with increasing levels of hCG, which peak between 8 and 11 weeks, a common time for nausea or vomiting to be at its worst.

Other theories point to the increase of the hormones progesterone and estrogen, which can lead to food aversions and an increased sense of smell that turns you off some favourite foods or even makes you nauseated. I have known some hard-core coffee drinkers who, once they've become pregnant, are so sickened by the smell of coffee that they don't want to touch a cup until after the baby is born. Vegetarians may suddenly like the smell of meat and crave steak and hamburgers, and some fish lovers can no longer stand to have fish cooked in the house. Situations like these may last the duration of your pregnancy but often improve after your first trimester.

Good Reasons for Grazing

Although eating is probably the last thing you feel like doing, it will honestly help the nausea. Eating small, regular meals is crucial to being able to enjoy *any* food during this time. Having a little of what you feel like—a cracker, some dry cereal, or fruit—may help ease the nausea. When it subsides, take the opportunity to eat a super-nutritious meal to maximize your nutrient intake while you can. Be sure to include a good source of protein at each meal, as it helps alleviate the nausea better than carbohydrates do.

Eating before bed may also help, since it's a long time between your last meal of the day and breakfast the next morning. Blood sugar can easily become too low during this time, causing nausea upon rising. Shortly before bedtime, try to eat a fairly significant snack of complex carbohydrates and protein, such as oatmeal made with almond, goat's, or cow's milk. The protein from the milk will help slow down the release of the complex carbohydrates, providing a more steady blood sugar level through the night. Even waking up in the middle of the night and grabbing a little extra snack may help.

When you wake up in the morning, try to eat before getting out of bed, and wait about 15 to 20 minutes before becoming upright, to allow time for your blood sugar level to rise. Try a carbohydrate-rich cracker or a handful of your favourite dry cereal—anything that can sit by your bedside all night without spoiling. If these don't work, experiment with other foods until you find something that does the trick.

Tips for Tricky Tummies

- Eat something small every two hours. Include snacks of protein-rich foods (see the box), which help to balance blood sugar levels much better than eating carbohydrate-rich foods on their own.
- Avoid coffee and sugary or refined foods. They will fill you up on empty calories and have no nutritional value. When you can eat, make it count.
- Between meals, drink plenty of water, diluted juice, or herbal tea. Drinking lots of liquid with a meal may make you feel worse.
- Avoid fatty, fried, and spicy foods. Fatty foods take longer to digest and may leave you feeling unwell, even on a good day.
- Try ginger tea. Ginger is known as a digestive soother and in some cases can help ease nausea. You can make your own by grating some fresh ginger into a cup of hot water. Sip this throughout the day.

Good Sources of Protein

Animal meats: poultry, beef, and pork*
Fish and seafood*
Eggs and dairy*
Beans, peas, and lentils
Nuts and nut butters, seeds
Tofu and tempeh
Quinoa*
Amaranth
Buckwheat
Spirulina*
Hemp seeds*
Whey,* rice, and hemp* protein powder
Chia, or Salba (known as a superfood, this seed is ground and can be added to foods such as yogurt, baking, and smoothies. Available at health food stores.)*

* A complete protein containing all the essential amino acids.

- Look for wristbands that are used for travel or sea sickness. They work by pressing on an acupressure point on the underside of your wrist. You can find them at most pharmacies.
- Take 100 to 200 milligrams (mg) of vitamin B6 in the pyridoxal-5-phosphate (P5P) form daily in divided doses. Vitamin B6 helps your liver to eliminate excess hormones and may alleviate your nausea. *Note:* Do not take this level of vitamin B6 while breastfeeding, as it may decrease breast milk production.
- Homeopathic preparations and tissue salts are usually quite successful too. Consult a naturopath or homeopath for specific remedies.

THE SCOOP ON MOM-TO-BE SUPPLEMENTS

Prenatal Multinutrient

Ideally, you began taking a multivitamin and mineral before conceiving. If not, your obstetrician, doctor, or midwife (and any other health practitioner) will likely advise you to take a

> ### Healthy Super-Snacks
>
> Veggie sticks with dip: hummus or bean dip, baba ganoush, yogurt dip
>
> Celery, banana, or apple with almond butter
>
> Smoothies: banana, frozen berries, ground flax, milk of choice, hemp or rice protein powder (used together or on their own), flax oil, almond butter
>
> Brown rice cakes with almond and apple butter or hummus
>
> Organic plain yogurt mixed with fruit or applesauce with granola
>
> Dried fruit (organic/unsulphured) with nuts and seeds and whole grain cereal
>
> Baked organic tortilla chips with hummus and salsa
>
> Low-sodium pretzels or crackers with bean dip
>
> Hard-boiled egg with fruit
>
> Cheddar or cottage cheese with crackers or fruit
>
> Protein bar or dried fruit and nut bar such as Lärabar
>
> Low-sugar whole grain or granola bars with at least 4 grams (g) protein

prenatal vitamin for the duration of your pregnancy and while breastfeeding. If they don't, I strongly recommend that you start taking one now. Your baby will take from you what she needs, and you might become deficient in certain nutrients, even if you're eating a good diet. Your body's requirements for certain vitamins and minerals increase well above your usual dietary intake. And as I mentioned earlier, influencing the development of your baby with key nutrients such as folic acid and B12, vitamin D, DHA, calcium and magnesium, zinc, and iron may have lifelong benefits in decreasing the risk of heart disease, diabetes, osteoporosis, learning difficulties, hyperactivity, and developmental delays.

When choosing a prenatal multivitamin, make sure it's good quality and has high absorbability. Cheaper supplements are often in a hard tablet form, with the nutrients bound in a way that is difficult to digest and absorb. For example, the calcium found in the most common brand of pregnancy vitamin, Materna, is in the carbonate form. This type of calcium, known as a "salt," isn't as readily absorbed and utilized by our bodies. It's considered a cheap form of calcium and is commonly used in less expensive multivitamins. Try to avoid prenatal vitamins with "calcium carbonate" on the label and look, instead, for those with the "citrate/malate," "fumarate," or "amino acid chelate" form of calcium and magnesium—this form is more absorbable, offering close to 70 percent absorbability of the value on the bottle. Usually capsules, as opposed to hard tablets, contain more absorbable nutrients. Vitamin D should be in the D3 form and zinc in the same form as calcium above.

Wherever you live, I would highly recommend visiting a good health food or supplement store to find the most bio-available (meaning that your body can absorb it easily) pre- and postnatal multinutrient. With your baby taking what he needs from your bones, brain, and storage sites such as your liver, a very absorbable multi will make it easier for your body to digest and assimilate these nutrients. You can speak with your nutritionist or naturopath for recommended products. Also check out the resource section at the end of the book for my recommendations.

> ### From the Mouths of Moms
>
> I started taking my multivitamin after my doctor confirmed my pregnancy, and I found it really hard to get down. I was feeling so nauseated, and when I did take it, I ended up constipated. I was worried about not taking it, because my doctor said it was important. So I kept taking it and ended up getting hemorrhoids from being constipated. I asked around, as some of my friends had just had babies, to see what they took and found a great alternative at a supplement store that didn't affect me in the same way. I couldn't go on like that, and it was only the beginning of my pregnancy!
>
> —SUZIE, MOM OF ADISON

Folic Acid

Folic acid is a synthetic vitamin that decreases the risk of neural tube defects (NTDs) such as spina bifida and other birth abnormalities, including congenital heart disease, urinary tract problems, oral facial clefts, limb defects, and some pediatric cancers. When found in food, the vitamin is called folate; folate-rich foods include dark-green leafy vegetables, beans, chickpeas, lentils, wheat germ, nuts, and seeds. Yet folate is surprisingly not as absorbable as synthetic folic acid.

The Society of Obstetricians and Gynaecologists of Canada (SOGC) and the Motherisk Program at the Hospital for Sick Children in Toronto concluded in recent research that folic acid supplementation during pregnancy can dramatically reduce these types of birth defects.[1]

A recent study in Canada found a 43 percent decrease in NTDs after cereal products were fortified with folic acid, even without the mothers taking a daily folic acid supplement.[2] Under the best scenario, pregnant women will take a daily folic acid supplement for at least three months before conceiving. Taking a daily level of 400 micrograms (mcg), or 0.4 milligrams (mg) to 1000 mcg, or 1 mg, before you conceive or as soon as you know you're pregnant also reduces the risk of premature delivery by 70 percent.[3] A higher level of folic acid, at 5000 mcg (5 mg), is recommended only in certain circumstances, such as when the mother-to-be has diabetes, has a family history of NTDs, is obese, or had a poor diet from three months prior to and 12 weeks following conception. Folic acid at the 400 to 1000 mcg level should be taken during pregnancy and beyond to breastfeeding. Most prenatal multivitamins have this level already, but double-check. If your multi doesn't contain this amount, top it up with an additional folic acid supplement.

> ### More Reason to Take Your Vitamins
>
> Taking a prenatal multivitamin and mineral that contains folic acid, rather than just taking folic acid on its own, has been shown to be even more beneficial for many aspects of good health for your baby now and later in life.

The Wonder Brain Supplement: DHA

You may have heard of omega-3 fatty acids, EPA, DHA, fish oils, or other similar terms describing good or essential fats. Well, docosahexaenoic acid (DHA, for short) is the most important of the omega-3 or omega-6 polyunsaturated fatty acids (PUFAs) when it comes to pregnancy. In recent years, awareness of the importance of all essential fatty acids (EFAs) has increased, and this is a good time to understand why they're essential for you and your developing baby.

Taking two types of omega-3 fatty acids, EPA and DHA, during pregnancy and while breastfeeding has far-reaching benefits that will be seen not only during baby's first years, but throughout life. While pregnant, you can take a mix of EPA and DHA in supplement form, but you want to make sure that the level of DHA is high enough (see below). DHA is crucial during pregnancy and breastfeeding because it

- provides the fuel for baby's developing brain and retina, improving visual acuity (clear vision);
- increases cognitive function, intelligence, and IQ;
- reduces the risk of attention deficit/hyperactivity disorder (ADD/ADHD), dyslexia, dyspraxia, and other developmental disorders;
- increases gestation time and birth weight (this is a good thing, even though you may want your baby out sooner by the end of the third trimester!); and
- may reduce the severity of allergies.

Furthermore, DHA deficiency has been strongly linked with postnatal depression, poor concentration and memory, and learning difficulties in the pre- and postnatal period for mom.

DHA is stored in your brain and tissues as well as in your red blood cells (RBCs). In an amazing process, the placenta takes what you have in your blood and directs it to the baby as needed. It can take up to eight weeks for DHA to accumulate in your red blood cells in high enough levels for it to be passed along to your baby, so start taking it early and continue throughout pregnancy and breastfeeding. As your pregnancy progresses, you may experience forgetfulness or a lack of concentration, both commonly referred to as "pregnancy brain." These can be signs of DHA deficiency as the DHA in your brain (especially if there isn't enough in your RBCs) is nabbed by "you know who"—your baby.

For vegetarian or vegan moms-to-be, who are commonly deficient in DHA, finding a way to meet your requirements through algae or fish sources will avoid your deficiency being passed along to your baby and lessen the risks described above.

Since attending a conference a few years ago given by Dr. Nigel Plummer—a prominent biochemist from the United Kingdom who specializes in the use of fish oils and probiotics—I have followed his recommendation of advising levels of 1200 mg of DHA daily during the first and second trimesters and have seen hundreds of moms feel the benefits. They experience much less forgetfulness, or "mommy brain," after the baby is born and have better concentration. In his lecture, Dr. Plummer explained that countries with the lowest incidence of postnatal depression, such as Japan, eat an amount of fish similar to this level. Because women in these countries eat a diet high in oily fish most of their lives, they have higher amounts of DHA in their bodies and may not need to supplement as much to maintain that level. Here in North America we are typically deficient in DHA, and you would need to eat about 3 pounds of wild salmon, mackerel, sardines, or herring daily to match 1200 mg of DHA. That's a lot of fish!

If you suffer from pregnancy sickness, you may not be able to tolerate this amount until the sickness subsides. Taking DHA in a pill form (at close to 600 mg) may be the best option at this point, while still trying to eat some wild-caught oily fish.

Probiotics: The Good Bugs

Probiotics, acidophilus, bifidus, and live cultures are names given to good or beneficial bacteria that live in our small and large intestines. Believe it or not, you have 100,000 billion of what I like to call "good guys" in your intestines. They offer health benefits that are still being researched. Good guys are also found on the surface of the skin and in the urethra, vagina, and respiratory tract. The most common types are *Lactobacillus acidophilus* and *Bifidobacterium*. We carry about 1.5 pounds of bacteria in our bodies, with between 33 and 50 percent found in our stool. There are about 500 types of bacteria in the digestive tract (small and large intestine), a lot of them not known to even the best researchers. Bacteria generally get a bad rap as we strive to keep a "clean" environment. However, the good guys living in us actually keep us healthier and stronger and support the immune system to deal with unwanted bacteria, such as *Bacteroides, Clostridium, Enterobacteria,* and *E. coli*. During the 17th European Congress on Obesity, a researcher presented findings that showed probiotics helped to reduce the risk of obesity one year after birth.[4]

Taking a probiotics supplement is the best way to colonize the intestines with these good guys. Eating plain organic yogurt is also beneficial (sweetened yogurt reduces the number of beneficial bacteria), but you won't get the same numbers as in a good-quality supplement. Especially if you have taken antibiotics recently, a potent probiotics is essential. Levels of over three billion bacteria should be taken daily of two or more strains of good bacteria—more with symptoms of yeast or thrush, gassiness, diarrhea, or constipation. See the Resources for reputable supplement companies offering probiotics.

Calcium and Vitamin D

Calcium and vitamin D, along with magnesium and phosphorus, help to build strong bones. Your baby will accumulate about 30 g (30,000 mg) of calcium during your pregnancy taken from you, about 80 percent of it in the third trimester.[6] Supplementing calcium at that stage is highly recommended (see the table on page 50 in Chapter 3 for specific amounts). In your first trimester, the amount given in your prenatal multivitamin should be enough for now if you're eating a diet including calcium-rich foods (see the resource section for food sources).

Benefits of Good Bacteria in the Digestive System

Good bacteria

- manufacture B vitamins for energy and many important cell functions and vitamin K for blood clotting;
- reduce the possibility of allergies and related conditions of asthma and eczema by 50 percent when a probiotics supplement with *Lactobacillus* and *acidophilus* strains is taken;[5]
- fight off bacteria that can cause sickness such as food poisoning (*E. coli*, *Salmonella*);
- are extremely important for overall health of both mom and baby, as over 80 percent of the immune system is linked to the digestive system;
- help avoid digestive issues such as gassiness, constipation, diarrhea, and irritable bowel diseases;
- alleviate colic symptoms in your baby;
- have powerful anti-tumour potential;
- aid in the digestion of food;
- help protect against leaky gut (see Chapter 6); and
- increase the absorption of calcium, magnesium, and iron (especially in formula-fed babies).

Vitamin D supplementation has been linked to a decreased risk of preeclampsia, type 1 diabetes, asthma, and schizophrenia, and to improved growth and bone strength. If you are deficient in vitamin D, your baby may be also.

Vitamin D, calcium, and magnesium all need to be taken together for maximum absorption of these bone-building nutrients.

Foods (and Other Things) to Steer Clear Of

During pregnancy it's important to avoid certain foods that carry a higher risk of making you sick and thus harming your developing baby. Your immune army is suppressed, known as "down regulation," leaving you more susceptible to bacteria and viruses. And some bacteria and parasites have potential life-threatening consequences for the fetus.

- Raw eggs and poultry are a potential source of *Salmonella* bacteria. Make sure that eggs are cooked until solid (sorry, no more sunny side up) and avoid mayonnaise made with raw eggs. When cooking chicken, be sure the internal temperature reaches 82°C (180°F) and reheated chicken reaches 74°C (165°F).
- Pâté and soft and blue cheeses are commonly unpasteurized and may be contaminated with *Listeria* (known to cause miscarriage). Avoid Brie, Camembert, Stilton, Roquefort, soft goat or sheep cheese, and feta.
- Raw shellfish and sushi may contain parasites, which aren't good for anyone, but especially pregnant women—symptoms can be similar to serious food poisoning. Enjoy vegetarian sushi as an alternative.
- Deli meats not only contain nitrates, but may contain *Listeria* as well. If you do eat deli or lunch meat, it must be reheated thoroughly. However, it's better to avoid deli meat altogether—studies show that nitrate-rich foods, such as hot dogs, bacon, and lunch meat, contain potential cancer-forming nitrosamines.
- Fish that's high in mercury is known to be a neurotoxin and so can be very harmful to baby's developing nervous system. Avoid tuna, shark, swordfish, king mackerel, orange roughy, tilefish, marlin, and all farmed fish, including salmon. Get to know your local fishmonger, who can suggest wild varieties to enjoy a few times a week.

- Green or sprouted potatoes should be avoided. Research is divided over whether the solanine present in green and sprouting potatoes poses harmful effects to the baby.
- Liver intake should be limited or avoided altogether. High levels of vitamin A (retinol) are potentially unsafe for the fetus. Liver is also the detoxification organ, and depending on the animal's diet, medications, and hormone administration, you may be eating the toxins and waste products the liver was trying to break down.
- Caffeine found in coffee, soft drinks, black and green tea, yerba mate, guarana, and, to a lesser amount, chocolate (sorry!) should be eliminated from your diet. No amount of caffeine is good for a developing baby. Caffeine can cross the placental barrier, and although your liver is able to break it down and detoxify it, your baby is less able to. Caffeine is a stimulant, has diuretic effects (leading to a loss of fluid), increases heart and breathing rates, and may be associated with miscarriage, premature birth, and low birth weight. Decaffeinated coffee, unfortunately, isn't much better. It still contains two stimulants, as well as the chemicals used in the decaffeination process. If you're a die-hard coffee drinker and can't live without your daily cup of joe, Swiss Water Process decaffeinated coffee, which uses fewer chemicals, is your best option. But do be aware that even decaffeinated coffee contains some caffeine.
- Alcohol is strictly off-limits during pregnancy and even while breastfeeding. Alcohol is a big anti-nutrient, meaning that it uses up a lot of nutrients when it's broken down and supplies nothing in return. It can reach the baby through the bloodstream and is detrimental to the development of his brain and organs. There's really no safe time to consume alcohol, as so much is going on each and every day of your pregnancy. Alcohol can also cause fetal alcohol spectrum disorder, which can mean a host of difficulties for a child, including developmental delays, social difficulties, and physical disabilities. And there's no conclusive safe limit of alcohol consumption. It's just not worth it. Stop drinking alcohol as soon as your pregnancy test is positive, if not before.
- Drugs and cigarettes are also off-limits. Some over-the-counter medications may be unsafe during pregnancy, so be sure to speak with your doctor or midwife to clarify what is safe. Motherisk is an excellent online resource for what you can and can't take during pregnancy and while breastfeeding (www.motherisk.org).

- Fruits and vegetables need to be washed thoroughly to ensure that all the soil and possible contaminants are removed. Toxoplasmosis, a parasitic disease, may be in the soil that fruits and vegetables are grown in and even in your own backyard, so be sure to wear gloves when gardening and to cover any cuts where this parasite may get into your blood. Cats are common hosts, so if you have a cat, ask someone else to change the cat litter (finally!), and avoid being scratched.
- Genetically modified (GM) foods have been changed from their natural state by manually altering their DNA. Adding a gene from another organism to a tomato, soybean, canola plant, or corn seed alters the structure and DNA of that food, and our bodies are unsure what to do with it. Although research on eating GM food during pregnancy is limited, what we do know about it isn't looking good. For the sake of your developing baby, try to stay away from GM crops, including nonorganic soy, corn, canola, and cotton—they may be the cause of a new "something" in years to come. And remember that although you may not eat these foods, they're fed to livestock and so are part of your meat, and many packaged foods, even chocolate bars, also contain GM ingredients.

Eating Organic and Avoiding Genetically Modified Food

Thousands of chemicals are found in the food chain, many of them from pesticides and herbicides. These chemicals can be toxic to our bodies, but they are especially so for the developing baby. After I found out that pesticides and herbicides were detected in the umbilical cord, I was so thankful that I had eaten organic as much as possible (although not 100 percent) during my pregnancies. It's not always financially possible to eat entirely organic, but do what you can. Any organic is better than none.

Organic food has become increasingly popular over the years and continues to grow more mainstream. In 2009, Canada enacted the *Organic Products Regulations,* which allow consumers to be confident when purchasing organics, whether fresh foods or mixed products containing many ingredients. For a farm to be certified organic, specific protocols need to be followed. Rather than herbicides and pesticides, preventative insect- and disease-controlling methods must be used. The use of synthetic chemicals or feeds (for livestock, which also must be fed organic feed), antibiotics, growth enhancers, hormones, colouring or artificial additives, ionizing radiation, or genetically engineered plants or animals is strictly forbidden. Farmers first must apply to a certifying body for an inspection and then grow their crops or raise their livestock according to organic standards for 36 months before they can call themselves "certified organic."[7] The Ontario Ministry of Agriculture, Food and Rural Affairs explains, "Food products labelled as organic must contain at least 95% organic ingredients (not including water and salt). The individual organic ingredients can be listed on the label when at least 70% of the product ingredients are organic."[8] Certified organic food is also a safe way to avoid GMO food. If a food is genetically modified, it can't be classed as organic.

See the "Shopper's Guide to Pesticides" on page 149 for a list of produce that's sprayed less and so isn't as important to buy organic.

HALFWAY THERE: THE SECOND TRIMESTER

By the time you reach your second trimester, you're probably not as tired, and the morning sickness has subsided. If you haven't already been able to take your multivitamin and extra vitamin D, calcium, magnesium, probiotics, and DHA, start now and continue until you finish breastfeeding (see the table on page 57 for specific amounts).

Your baby now has developing hormonal glands, transparent skin, ears, and bones and bone marrow. The lungs, liver, and immune system are continuing to form. Now that you're

From the Mouths of Moms

When I found out I was pregnant, I immediately had a ferocious appetite. I guess it was those hormones. I could eat all day, and did, for the most part. I managed to eat even when I was nauseated. Ice cream was my weakness—it was a hot summer, and it went down so easily. I ended up putting on 65 pounds throughout my pregnancy. I couldn't believe how tired I was all the time—I had no energy, and I was depressed about being so big. The doctor was worried about gestational diabetes, which I had never heard of, and he was right to be. After a glucose tolerance test, I was diagnosed with gestational diabetes. I had to have many more ultrasounds and ended up in the hospital with an obstetrician instead of my midwife at home for the labour. I still have 20 pounds to lose, and my baby is now one year old. It was easier and more fun putting on the weight than it has been getting it off!

—SARAH, MOM OF HANNAH

feeling better, this is the time to concentrate on improving your diet to keep up with nutrient demand on your body as your baby grows.

Continue to eat small meals throughout the day since your stomach is slowly being squished in your abdomen as the baby takes up more space. Eating regularly will also help keep your blood sugar in balance, lessening the chance of mood swings, lack of energy, and tiredness. And eating a balanced diet can prevent gestational diabetes and dramatic weight gain.

MAKING EVERY MOUTHFUL COUNT

Although some see pregnancy as a licence to eat whatever they want, since they're going to put on weight anyway, try to be a bit reserved when it comes to treating yourself. What you eat provides the nourishment for your developing baby, and although it tastes good, the fat and sugar found in ice cream aren't essential for her growth! The average weight gain during your pregnancy should be between 30 and 35 pounds (14 to 16 kg), although I have seen many women with higher weight gain. Putting on too much weight may increase your risk of pregnancy complications, such as gestational diabetes, pre-eclampsia, and water retention. That said, dieting to avoid gaining much weight may put your baby at risk for preterm labour, low birth weight, and a host of potentially lifelong diseases and

Sweeping Statements

This wasn't strange advice, but it was very disheartening. I gained 45 pounds while pregnant. I had a couple of early growth spurts, and my family doctor kept telling me I was gaining far too much weight and had to stop eating so much. I promptly switched to midwifery care, and my midwife was awesome. She tested me for gestational diabetes twice and then did some ultrasounds, and we found out that I was having a very large baby. Finding out if there's a reason for weight gain is imperative. My family doctor had me feeling really down and worried, but my midwife said, "Don't worry; keep doing what you're doing. Your baby is healthy, and that's all that matters."
—JENNIFER, MOM OF ONE. (She went on to have a healthy 11 pound, 5 ounce baby by Caesarean section.)

developmental problems. Pregnancy is often hard enough without these extra concerns.

Avoid or limit high-fat foods such as french fries, potato chips, red meat, and cheese, which are high in saturated fats and have more calories than protein or carbohydrates. Each gram of protein or carbohydrate provides 4 calories, but every gram of fat gives you 9 calories, meaning that you're doubling your calories when eating a fat-rich food. When you eat fat, make sure that a large percentage of it is an essential fat (EFA).

Allergic Parents = Allergic Child?

Limiting or avoiding foods that mom or dad is allergic to may reduce the chance of your baby reacting to the same foods or to new ones either in breast milk or when the baby starts solids. If mom is allergic to a food, there is a 40 percent chance that baby will be allergic, and a 60 percent chance if both mom and dad are allergic. The allergy may not be to the same foods, but the allergic potential is higher.

There's actually no need to eat any more than before you were pregnant until you're closer to your third trimester, when an increase of 200 calories per day is needed. Once your baby is born and you're breastfeeding, you'll need an extra 500 calories per day. But remember that quality is more important than quantity. If you're not eating foods that offer vital vitamins and minerals, you and your baby may become nutrient deficient. Try to eat the following foods every day:

- five pieces of colourful fruit, such as apple, banana, pear, melon, berries, kiwi, citrus, mango, papaya, or grapes;
- two green vegetables, such as spinach, kale, broccoli, beans, peas, chard, zucchini, cucumber, lettuce, watercress, arugula, or sunflower sprouts;
- two other colourful vegetables, for example, peppers, cauliflower, squash, and sweet potato;

From the Mouths of Moms

I relied on muffins for both of my pregnancies. In the nesting phase, I made a bunch and froze them—they were easily taken out when needed. I tried to make them nutritious by throwing in flax, nuts, bran, raisins, and bananas—but the odd time they had to have some chocolate chips in them to satisfy my sweet tooth!
—SYLVIA, MOM OF TWO

- protein from eggs, meat, poultry, fish, lentils, beans, hard cheese, cottage cheese, nuts, and seeds;
- carbohydrate-rich foods from whole grains, including brown rice, quinoa, whole wheat, spelt, kamut, millet, and oats, in the form of bread, pasta, cooked grain, or cereal; and
- essential fatty acids (EFAs) from flax seeds or oil; hemp seeds or oil; almonds, walnuts, Brazil nuts, and hazel nuts; sunflower, sesame, and pumpkin seeds; and oily fish such as wild salmon, herring, mackerel, and sardines.
- To balance your meals, think about dividing your plate in half. One half should be fruits and vegetables, one quarter of the remaining side

should be protein, and the last quarter should come from carbohydrate-rich foods. Nuts and seeds make excellent snacks combined with fruit or can be sprinkled on salads and vegetables.

> ## Good-for-You Fish
>
> The following fish choices are high in omega-3 fats and low in contaminants:
>
> Anchovy
> Atlantic mackerel
> Atlantic pollock (Boston bluefish)
> Capelin
> Char
> Hake
> Herring
> Lake whitefish
> Mullet
> Rainbow trout
> Salmon
> Sardines
> Smelt
>
> *Source:* Health Canada, "Mercury in Fish," www.hc-sc.gc.ca/fn-an/securit/chem-chim/environ/mercur/cons-adv-etud-eng.php.

ON THE HOME STRETCH: THE THIRD TRIMESTER

By your third trimester, you'll have gotten used to being kicked and punched, and you may feel as though Junior is never going to make an appearance. Sleeping becomes difficult; leg cramps, heartburn, and visiting the toilet more often than you ever thought possible all become regular parts of your day. But the end is in sight!

Your baby is starting to pack on the pounds as he stores fat to keep warm after birth. All bones are developed, although they are not hard and strong like ours—yet. Baby is starting to store calcium, vitamin D, iron, zinc, and phosphorus to be used for so many important functions after birth. At week 37 your baby is full

Sweeping Statements

Pregnancy myth: One woman advised me not to work at any tasks that put my arms above my head because the cord would knot or wrap around the baby's neck.
—DIANE, MOM OF THREE

term and can be born at any time without preterm complications. However, although you are more than likely ready for your baby to make an appearance, the longer he stays in you, the healthier he'll likely be. During these last few weeks of pregnancy, your baby's systems continue to develop, including the important immune system. Your baby is receiving antibodies to protect him from infection as he crosses the placenta. And more antibodies will come from colostrum and breast milk after birth.

At this point, you can start to increase the amount of food in your diet, but not by too much. Only an extra 200 calories per day are needed—the equivalent of half an avocado and a small sprinkling of sunflower seeds on top of your spinach salad (because I know you already had salad on the menu!), or one hard-boiled egg, a slice of rye bread, and half a cup of blueberries. Not quite the all-you-can-eat buffet you might have imagined! If you try to keep to this amount, your body will go back to its pre-pregnancy weight much faster after the baby is born. If your weight has crept up more than you had hoped, try to be sensible about your eating habits (I know, I know—cravings aren't always for broccoli and bananas). Remember that your diet is providing your baby with the nutrients he needs for healthy growth, lessening the chances of adult diseases.

Make a habit of eating breakfast every day. Smoothies are a favourite of mine, not only for breakfast but at any time of day: They're quick and easy and can be packed with all sorts of essential nutrients. If you can't get your daily 2400 mg of DHA past your lips (see below), put it in here, or throw in greens such as spinach. Blend ground flax seeds and oil, protein (hemp, rice, or whey), and three servings of fruit, and you've got the healthiest meal in a glass. Have some frozen fruit on hand for those days when you didn't make it out shopping, and experiment to find your favourite combinations. See pages 35 and 245 for recipe suggestions.

Start to make extra food at dinner for the next day's lunch. A leftover chicken breast or piece of fish with a salad makes a fantastic lunch. Thinking ahead will help you eat well and avoid mealtime stress.

MORE BRAINY DHA

As you enter your third trimester, increase your DHA intake to 2400 mg per day. This additional DHA supports the rapid development of your baby's brain and retinas. It will also lessen the possibility of postpartum depression and pregnancy or mommy brain. Maintain this level until baby is three months old if breastfeeding. If you end up formula-feeding, go back to 600 to 1200 mg per day to replenish what your baby has taken. Be sure to read the label of your supplement, as most capsules only contain 100 to 200 mg. Fish oil or DHA in a liquid form usually yields higher amounts than capsules, so one teaspoon might equal 6 to 12 pills. If you're vegetarian or vegan, you may already be deficient in DHA from avoiding fish. DHA products from algae sources are available, but note that typically they provide only 100 to 200 mg of DHA per capsule. See the Resources for recommendations.

MORE GOOD BACTERIA

Now is the time to increase your intake of probiotics to enhance your immune system and colonize the birth canal with millions of good bacteria for your baby's journey into the world. Your body will redirect *Lactobacillus acidophilus* from your intestines to the birth canal, where your baby will be exposed to it during delivery. This exposure or inoculation of beneficial bacteria during vaginal births gives your baby an important boost of immunity before she enters our world of bacteria after being in the sterile environment of the womb. It may also reduce the risk of allergies. If you haven't taken any probiotics yet, a very high dose is needed to get the good bacteria in quickly (but start slowly to avoid excess gassiness). If you're already taking probiotics, double your dose. It may be more cost-effective to find a stronger product than take more of what you have.

Help for Heartburn

Heartburn doesn't affect every pregnant woman, but most do experience it. The increase of estrogen can weaken your esophageal hiatus muscle, leading to heartburn and even vomiting. Eating little and often should help—it's not like there's much room for a big meal in there anyway. Avoid spicy, rich, fatty, tomato-based foods, as well as caffeine, chocolate, sugar, and citrus fruits.

Try to leave three hours between your last meal and bed, making sure that you sit upright until bedtime. You may find that lying propped up on an extra pillow helps ease the symptoms. A calcium and magnesium liquid supplement can soothe your heartburn and give you the calcium and magnesium that your body needs (see the Resources for recommended supplements). Taking vegetarian digestive enzymes after a meal might help too. Although most people reach for antacids, some research suggests that there may be a link between taking antacids while pregnant and creating the potential for baby to develop asthma and allergies later on.[9] This may be something to discuss further with your nutritionist or naturopath, doctor, or midwife.

Coping with Sleepless Nights

Sleepless nights may be Mother Nature's way of preparing you for life with a newborn, but she should really give you a break and let you sleep for the last month or two of your pregnancy. Your mind is racing, the baby is doing gymnastics as soon as you crawl under the covers, heartburn or cramps are keeping you up, and you're just downright uncomfortable. Taking calming minerals of calcium and magnesium before bed should help you fall asleep faster and get you back to sleep more easily (and also helps build strong bones and teeth). Taking 1000 mg of calcium and 500 mg of magnesium combined, preferably in the liquid carbonate form, before bed should do the trick (and may calm heartburn, as well).

A warm bath with Epsom salts (magnesium sulphate) is soothing and beneficial for sleep as well as for relaxed muscles.

EASING LEG CRAMPS

Painful is the only way to describe leg cramps. They are usually due to a nutritional imbalance or deficiency or to changes in your circulation that come with carrying the extra weight. Try to increase calcium- and potassium-rich foods, including bananas (which also contain tryptophan that will help you sleep). Almonds, wild salmon, sardines, sesame seeds and tahini, yogurt, and cottage cheese should all be regulars in your diet. Heat also helps alleviate cramps—try a hot water bottle on your leg cramp (but never over your abdomen), or flex your foot if the cramp is in your leg.

Now you're all set to sit back and wait for the big appearance! Good luck, and see you on the other side of labour.

Before-Birth Checklist

- Look into hiring a lactation consultant or a postpartum doula.
- Stock up on freezer meals and pantry essentials. Ask parents, in-laws, and other family and friends to make freezable dishes that will keep your eating on track after the baby comes. If you don't have anyone to help out, make a list of catering companies that will deliver fresh or frozen meals.
- Buy probiotics for you and your baby.
- Read the chapters on breastfeeding and formula-feeding to prepare yourself for nourishing your newborn.
- Jot down the phone numbers and websites for important resources: your doctor or pediatrician; your local breastfeeding clinic; Dr. Jack Newman's breastfeeding clinic, Newman Breastfeeding Clinic and Institute (www.ncbi.ca); La Leche League (www.lllc.ca); a nutritionist (www.sproutright.com), naturopath, homeopath, and osteopath; a local food-delivery service; a diaper service; your favourite takeout; a specialized baby store; and a nursing bra boutique.

2

NUTRITION FOR NEW MOMS
What You Need After Birth

After the long marathon of labour (for some, not all), it's important to replenish your energy stores with nutritious food. However, feeding yourself probably isn't high on your priority list, now that you have your new arrival to watch over, so get baby's dad, grandma, friends, or anyone who's willing to make you some healthy meals and snacks, and ask them to keep them coming. Breastfeeding mothers need more of certain nutrients to keep up with breast milk demands. Calorie intake should increase by 500 calories a day (for example, two tablespoons of hummus and carrot sticks with about 20 almonds or cashews and a 50 g piece of cheese) to produce enough breast milk for your baby without leaving you zapped of energy. You might be concerned about losing the pounds gained during pregnancy, but trust me, you'll still lose weight if you stick to that number.

It took nine months to put on your pregnancy weight, and it might take longer to lose it. Don't have too high expectations, and understand

Get Some Sleep

It's always said that you should nap while your baby is sleeping. Let's be realistic here. How is the laundry, tidying up, or dinner supposed to get done? Magic? If sleeping when the baby does were that easy, there would be no need to talk about the incredible sleep deprivation you go through after baby comes. Use his nap time, instead, to eat something healthy in peace, and then move on to other tasks.

that your body has changed. Now is not the time to diet, but you *can* watch what you eat. Eat healthily instead of indulging your cake or cookie craving, and the weight will come off slowly and steadily. Exercise is crucial for slowly shedding some pounds, and it also helps increase your energy and put you in a good mood. Plenty of fitness companies offer stroller fitness, indoor aerobics, and boot camp classes with baby in tow if you want faster results than waiting for your pre-pregnancy shape to return on its own.

In the weeks and months after your baby is born, sleep deprivation and a whole new routine that you're not always in charge of can throw off eating patterns, leaving breakfast to happen closer to lunch, lunch nearer to dinner, and dinner before you go to bed, if at all. Even with the best of intentions, feeding yourself and your family might just become another stress in your day.

KEY NUTRIENTS AND SUPPLEMENTS FOR THE EARLY DAYS

MULTINUTRIENTS

In an ideal world, we would all eat freshly picked fruits and vegetables, have a plentiful supply on hand of the most nutritious whole grain cereals and bread, eat only fresh-caught fish, buy naturally farmed and fed poultry and red meat ... and have it cooked for us! And while we're at it, somebody else would wash the dishes after dinner and fold the laundry while we try to get some sleep. Well, that just isn't reality. Maybe this is your first baby, and feeding yourself is at the bottom of your list of things to do. So where are you going to get the vitamins, minerals, proteins, carbohydrates, and fats you need? This is where a good-quality multinutrient comes in handy. Your baby took all the vitamins and minerals she needed from you while in utero—calcium, iron, zinc, and vitamin D, to name a few—and may have left you deficient. A multinutrient will help ensure that you're getting a base level of nutrients daily. Even if you do manage to eat a healthy, balanced diet, it's still hard for your body to keep up with the nutrient demands of making breast milk. If you're not breastfeeding, you still need three to six months to replenish the stores of minerals and fats that were nabbed from you during pregnancy.

When it comes to buying a good-quality multinutrient, what should you look for? First, I'd suggest finding a health food or supplement store or asking a nutritionist, homeopath, or naturopath what brands she likes and why. Although a few chain drugstores and big-box retailers might carry some higher-quality natural products and supplements, you won't get the same level of help. Always look for a multi in capsule rather than tablet form. Capsules typically break down more easily, leading to better vitamin and mineral absorption.

Here's a rundown of the key vitamins and minerals your body needs every day, along with their most important functions.

- Fat-soluble vitamins—vitamins A, D, E, and K. These vitamins all have different roles in the body, from supporting healthy mucous membranes to maintaining bone health, ensuring good heart functioning, and providing normal blood clotting. All of these vitamins are stored in the liver and fatty tissues of the body, and their absorption is helped by eating fat at the same time as taking a supplement. Excessive amounts of any fat-soluble vitamin can be toxic. Double-check with a naturopath or nutritionist for safe supplement levels.
- Water-soluble vitamins—B vitamins, including B1, B2, B3, B5, B6, B12, folic acid, biotin, and vitamin C. These are needed every day: they are taken into the body and used, and anything left over is then excreted (B2 is the one that makes your urine turn bright yellow). B vitamins are important for many functions in the body but are best known for supplying energy. Be careful not to take more B6 than what's in your multi while breastfeeding, as too much might lower your breast milk production. Vitamin C is also used for an incredible number of processes in the body but is perhaps recognized most often for its immune-boosting properties. Vitamin C has an antihistamine effect (great for treating allergies) and is needed for cardiovascular health and wound healing. It's used up quickly in times of stress, which, let's face it, most of us go through, so make sure you're getting enough—about 2000 mg per day is good (in divided doses—1000 mg with breakfast and 1000 mg another time in the day). If you're breastfeeding, you need all of these water-soluble vitamins in your diet or from your multinutrient to pass them into your breast milk.
- Macro minerals, or big minerals, including calcium, magnesium, phosphorus, potassium, and sodium. Calcium is well known for building strong bones but is also needed to maintain your body's alkaline balance (see "Strong Bones" on

page 47). Magnesium is important for muscles, bones, the immune system, blood sugar balance, stress busting, and heart function. Both calcium and magnesium are calming minerals—taking them before bed can ensure a good night's sleep. Calcium requires phosphorus to help absorption and contribute to bone and teeth strength, kidney and heart function, and nerve and muscle activity. Potassium is crucial for heart function, nerves, muscles, kidneys, and blood. And sodium, which has a bad reputation (as it's overused), is actually important for keeping fluid levels in the body just right as well as maintaining a healthy heart.

- Micro minerals or trace minerals, the most important being iron, zinc, manganese, chromium, and selenium. Micro minerals are needed in smaller amounts in our bodies than macro minerals. Iron is essential to the development and growth of babies and children, and is used in the production of hemoglobin and by the immune system. Zinc is another incredibly important mineral that's involved in over 300 enzyme processes in the body. It's used by the immune system; along with B6, it aids in hydrochloric acid production in the stomach for digesting proteins and carbohydrates; it helps wound healing; and it supports reproductive organ growth and development. Manganese is needed to make strong bones, synthesize fats and cholesterol, protect your body from free radical damage, and help with balancing blood sugar levels. Chromium works with manganese to balance blood sugar levels. Selenium is an important anticancer mineral, it helps the body use vitamin E, and it helps build healthy cell membranes.

All of the above vitamins and nutrients are available from a wide variety of foods, but to get enough you need to eat a varied diet every day—and that doesn't always happen. In addition, nonorganic or conventional food contains less nutrients than organic food. To keep up with the requirements of your body at this stage, you'll need to take a good-quality multinutrient and even add an extra 1000 to 2000 mg of vitamin C, 1200 mg of calcium, and 600 to 800 mg of magnesium per day. If your blood sugar balance is up and down (as most of the population's is), you'll need an additional 200 to 400 mcg of chromium daily. White spots on your fingernails indicate zinc deficiency; add about 20 mg of zinc every day until they fade. Supplements are really the only way to correct deficiencies. A nutritionist or naturopath can help you identify what you might be deficient in and advise you how to correct it.

DHA FOR MOMMY BRAIN

Forgetfulness, inability to concentrate, and, some days, forgetting where the car keys are *and* where you parked the car can be blamed on mommy brain (finally, a valid excuse!). The phenomenal development and growth rate of your baby's neurological system and brain from the third trimester until she's three months old while breastfeeding demands a higher level of DHA. The DHA stored in your brain and tissues passes through your bloodstream to your baby. Amazingly, your DHA reserves provide the fuel to make another brain and nervous system. So you deserve a break if you don't remember where the diapers went! Sleep deprivation compounds the problem, and while a full week of eight hours of sleep each night might improve your functioning, it still won't help with the deficiency of DHA in your brain.

DHA deficiency increases the chances of postnatal depression—in fact, low levels are linked to depressive disorders in any individual. Having a baby is transformational enough without the added risk of depression and even suicidal thoughts. Media attention has increasingly been directed to postnatal depression and its treatment with antidepressants, but I would love to hear whether DHA supplementation was talked about before the prescription was written.

DHA comes from the family of omega-3 fatty acids. The best source of dietary DHA is from oily fish: salmon, tuna, herring, mackerel, sardines, and trout. If you're not a fish eater, there are other ways to get this important nutrient. I have a friend who couldn't take the fish oil in a liquid form (which yields a much higher amount per teaspoon) that I had recommended, no matter where she put it—in a smoothie, in salad dressing, or down the hatch with her nose plugged. Instead, she ended up taking handfuls of EPA/DHA capsules every day. It was what she could manage, and, although this was a more expensive way to take it, she was pleased that she'd made the effort and commented many times that her mommy brain was significantly less with her second child than with her first, born five years earlier.

A vegetarian or vegan source of omega-3 and DHA is algae—after all, it's what fish eat to become such rich sources. Vegans and vegetarians have a hard time getting enough DHA into their diet and have to take handfuls of algae DHA, which typically comes in 100 to 200 mg capsules, to get the recommended 1200 mg per day. In a study measuring DHA levels in breast milk, mothers following vegetarian and vegan diets had 50 to 70 percent less than fish-eating moms.[10] Other sources of omega-3 fats that vegetarians and vegans could benefit from eating include walnuts and pumpkin, sunflower, flax, chia, and hemp seeds, but I wouldn't recommend relying only on these food sources during pregnancy or breastfeeding, as the body's ability to digest or break these fats down to DHA is poor.

You need 2400 mg of DHA daily from the third trimester until your baby is three months old while breastfeeding. After three months, you can reduce the amount to 1200 mg per day. If you're not breastfeeding, 1200 mg a day for the first three months should top up what was taken from you during pregnancy. The best way to take DHA is in a liquid oil, which usually yields a higher level—as mentioned above, most omega-3 capsules yield only about 100 to 200 mg. At least 600 mg per day should be taken for six months after baby weans (or after baby is three months old if you're formula-feeding—the higher level above helps to prevent postnatal depression) to renourish your brain and build up your stores of DHA if you plan to have more babies.

When choosing your omega-3 or DHA supplement, always first read the label to make sure that it contains DHA. If the omega-3 isn't broken down or predigested to DHA (look for a milligram amount on the label), your body will use up the omega-3 before it's broken down to DHA, leaving you deficient. As with a multinutrient, buy your DHA from a reputable supplement or health food store, and ask staff about the different products. Or ask your nutritionist or naturopath for her recommendation. Genestra is a brand that I've recommended for many years—I prefer its process of extracting the oils from fish. In Genestra's patented process, triglyceride (fat) bonds are not broken apart, making the DHA more absorbable. Nutra Sea and Nordic Naturals are also good brands. It's worth comparing the price versus yield of DHA in various products.

PROBIOTICS

Billions of bacteria, both good and bad, live within humans' digestive tracts or, more specifically, the intestines. For overall health, a strong immune system, and effective digestion and detoxification of what we ingest, we need high levels of good bacteria. To explain further, I often use the analogy of a backyard. Picture a lovely green, lush, healthy lawn with few or no weeds. In the intestines, the lovely lawn without many weeds is what we'd like to see along the lining of our intestines—an abundance of good bacteria creates a healthy colonic environment. When the weeds, or bad bacteria, take over, the environment changes, leading to a not-so-green-and-lush lawn, or suboptimal health. This healthy environment must be cared for by supporting the proliferation of good bacteria with supplements called probiotics.

> ### Do You Need More Good Bacteria?
>
> Think of how gassy you are, how smelly the bathroom is after you've had a bowel movement. Do you have symptoms of thrush? Do you have alternating diarrhea and constipation? Answering yes to any of these questions could mean that you need to get a huge boost of good bacteria from probiotics.

The benefits of a healthy digestive system and a strong population of good bacteria are far-reaching and include

- lessening the potential for allergies;
- protecting against the ill effects of bad bacteria taking residence in the gut;
- better digestion of sugars (lactose);
- creating B and K vitamins in the gut; and
- detoxifying and positively transforming many unsavoury substances, such as heavy metals of lead, mercury, and cadmium, and releasing helpful substances from foods that help to slow cancer growth.

Antibiotics, unfortunately, have a similar effect in your intestines as weed killer on a lawn. Although antibiotics are designed to kill the bad bacteria, or weeds, in your gut (or elsewhere in your body), a side effect is that they also destroy a large amount of the good bacteria. When the lush, green, healthy grass is destroyed, this is an opportune time for the weeds to take over. For instance, if you tested strep B positive before delivery, you would have been given antibiotics during labour to kill the strep B bacteria and keep them from harming your baby. Although both mom and baby have benefited from killing the strep B, the beneficial bacteria in mom's intestines as well as those that the baby would take from the birth canal may have been wiped out. The immune-boosting effects of the beneficial bacteria for the newborn are now deficient, allowing any unfriendly bacteria to proliferate. Researchers attribute the rise of allergies in the developed world partly to the overuse of antibiotics. With the well-known fact that an intestinal environment colonized with predominantly beneficial bacteria can help reduce the risk of allergies by a whopping 50 percent, taking probiotics is crucial for anyone who has been on antibiotics.

What Makes a Good Probiotic?

When you're looking to buy a probiotic, quality really does matter. A reputable company will have high standards for the manufacturing process as well as excellent quality control. When you are deciding on a probiotic, it's all about the numbers. How many billions of bacteria is it supplying? Which strains of bacteria are you getting? Is it a human strain of bacteria (much more effective for colonizing the gut)? Look for one that has *Lactobacillus acidophilus* and *Bifidobacterium bifidum* and/or *lactis* on the label along with HMF (human microflora), for starters. Probiotics for infants under one year of age should contain *Bifidobacterium infantis*. If you've just been on antibiotics, you need to take a super-powered probiotic to get 130 billion good bacteria per day for at least seven days after finishing the course of antibiotics. Look for a product containing fructo-oligosaccharides, a prebiotic that's fuel for the probiotics—here, you're not only colonizing the intestines but also supporting the probiotic's proliferation. If you're suffering from symptoms of thrush, a level of about 24 to 28 billion total bacteria a day should be your minimum, taken in divided doses. For overall health and to support your immune and digestive systems, anywhere between 9 and 12 billion per day is a good level. When you first start taking probiotics, you could experience

> ### From the Mouths of Moms
>
> After my baby was born, I was amazed at what I could do with one hand. I managed to eat pretty well while my newborn was occupying one arm—cereal, soup, veggies and dip, eggs and toast, fruit and yogurt. I could even make pasta and rice with one hand! After the first couple of weeks, I started planning better. I'd make pasta salad with tuna, veggies, and beans that could be eaten out of the fridge or other one-dish meals that would be ready to heat and eat. And in a pinch, some trail mix and a glass of milk would always do the trick.
> —JEN, MOM OF ONE

an increase in gassiness, perhaps a bit of diarrhea, or even constipation for the first three days. I suggest starting with lower amounts than those listed above, taking your probiotics after food (unless the label says otherwise), and taking them in the evening. If you're giving probiotics to your baby, start in the morning so that any gassiness won't cause discomfort and wake her up in the night.

Because probiotics are live bacteria, they should be purchased from the fridge and kept refrigerated at home. Some probiotics are shelf stable for several months, but you'll lose some of those good guys the longer they're kept out of the fridge. But do take your probiotics on holiday with you, even if they won't be refrigerated—it's better to take them and lose a few in your supplement than not take them at all.

See Chapter 7 for more information about probiotics for infants and the immune system and page 57 for a table listing the quantities of supplements, including probiotics, you need.

MOMMY MEALS

Some basic tips for the new mom:

- Drink plenty of water! Aim for over 2 litres (L) filtered water a day.
- If you're breastfeeding and think your baby may be reacting to something in your diet, keep a food diary of what you eat and drink. Write down the symp-

---

Don't Forget to Feed Yourself

As a new mom, you're probably lucky some days if you shower, brush your teeth, and get out of your PJs. Eating takes a back seat to caring for your bundle of joy. But if you're a breastfeeding mom, your nutritional requirements are higher than when you were pregnant. Feeding yourself is an extra task that you don't always have time for. Let's make it simple.

- If you can't eat full meals, eat nutritious snacks throughout the day.
- Raw fruits and vegetables are healthy and fast, with little prep time.
- When you cook, make larger batches to save for the next day's meals. For example, grill four chicken breasts instead of two and add some to your salad or wrap for lunch, or mix with some frozen vegetables and rice for the next night's stir-fry.
- Have some dried fruit on hand for a quick energy boost.
- Stock up on meals that freeze well for fast and easy dinners (with extra for leftovers).

See "Mommy Meals," below, for more suggestions.

toms your baby is experiencing. Look back over 24 hours in your diary to try to figure out what may be the problem.

- Eat three meals each day and two to three snacks. Try to eat something about every two and a half to three hours. Eating regularly will help keep your blood sugar and energy balanced.

> ### When You Wake Up
>
> Every morning, make a mug of hot water with a squeeze of lemon in it and drink it before you have anything else. It starts your digestion working and stimulates the kidneys and liver, improving overall good health and giving you extra energy.

- Make sure you eat protein at each snack and meal. Increase your protein intake at breakfast especially by eating eggs, cottage cheese, or protein powder in a smoothie. I like to mix hemp and rice protein together to get a high level of protein and extra omega-3s and fibre.
- Increase your intake of fruits and veggies. A handful of almonds with an apple is an excellent snack, giving you fibre, carbohydrate, protein, essential fats, and tons of nutrients.
- Be sure to have at least five servings of fruits and veggies every day.
- Watch the amount of wheat and dairy that you're eating. These are the two most common food sensitivities. Try to switch up the grains you eat from wheat to spelt, kamut, oats, rice, or quinoa. Add rice or almond milk to your smoothie for a change from dairy milk.

BREAKFAST

- A piece of fruit (fruit should always be a part of your breakfast—try to eat it first, as it's easier on your digestion)
- Smoothie made with rice, almond, or cow's milk (see the recipe below)
- Organic oatmeal with rice, almond, or cow's milk and ground nuts and seeds (flax, sunflower, or pumpkin) and fresh fruit such as blueberries or pear
- Granola with yogurt or milk of choice (check the granola's sugar content before buying)
- Cold cereal with nuts and seeds or an egg
- Poached or scrambled egg on toast (kamut, spelt, rice, or whole wheat bread) or in a wrap with veggies

- French toast with fresh fruit and agave syrup
- Cereal and a boiled egg
- Toast with almond butter and fruit spread (sweetened with fruit juice instead of sugar)
- Live organic yogurt (if tolerated) with fruit and ground or whole nuts and seeds

LUNCH OR DINNER

- Large mixed salad with nuts, seeds, fish, chicken, tofu, cottage cheese, or egg
- Sandwich or wrap with fish, chicken, egg, cheese, nut butter (almond butter is good), or hummus and sprouts
- Any other grains, such as buckwheat, quinoa, amaranth, or rice, with tofu, chicken, or fish and vegetables—cooked together in a saucepan or as a stir-fry
- Pasta with sauce and chicken meatballs (see the recipe on page 258)
- Baked potato topped with chili (see the recipe on page 250) or cottage cheese, fish, and corn
- Falafel with hummus and salad
- Chicken, fish, or meat with two colourful vegetables
- Mixed bean salad (chickpeas, kidney, cannellini) with green beans and corn, and a leafy green salad on the side
- Quesadilla (see the recipe on page 260)
- Soup with whole grain bread or crackers and hummus
- Egg and vegetable frittata with salad
- Mixed nuts or seeds on top of anything
- Beans or pulses, such as chickpeas and lentils, with salad or grains

SNACKS

- Spelt or kamut bread with nut butter and fruit spread
- Crudités (vegetable sticks) with nut butter, guacamole, hummus, nuts, or seeds
- Air-popped popcorn drizzled with olive oil, herbs, and spices with nuts or seeds

- Oatcakes, rice cakes, Ryvita crispbread, or crackers with hummus, tahini (sesame seed paste), cottage cheese, avocado dip, or dairy, goat's milk, or sheep's milk cheese
- Organic baked corn chips with hummus or salsa
- Low-sodium pretzels with bean dip or hummus
- Smoothie (see the recipe below)
- Fruit with nut butter, such as banana or apple with almond butter
- Granola bar or dried fruit bar such as Lärabar

Mom's Super-Powered Smoothie

This smoothie is nutrient packed for every member of the family. If you're pregnant or breastfeeding, add fish oil to get beneficial omega-3 fats and DHA to you and your baby. Switch up the fruits to include mango, peach, melon, or other berries for different nutrient profiles. The banana masks most flavours, so this is a great place to hide some of the not-so-favourite foods.

1 cup	milk of choice	250 mL
1 to 2	bananas	1 to 2
½ cup	frozen wild blueberries	125 mL
½	pear (core removed)	½
Handful	sunflower sprouts or spinach	Handful
1 tbsp	flax oil	15 mL
2 tbsp	hemp and/or rice protein	30 mL
1 tbsp	molasses (optional)	15 mL

1. Blend all ingredients in a blender until smooth. Serve immediately. Makes about 1½ cups (375 mL).

NUTRITIONAL INFORMATION
This smoothie is high in fibre, antioxidants, omega-3 fats, and protein to keep blood sugar stable.

NUTRITIONAL NUTS AND BOLTS
An In-Depth Look at the Nutrients Your New Baby Needs

Now that your baby has arrived, let's lay the groundwork for what you need to know about vitamins and minerals, fats, and oils in the first six months to a year of your baby's life. Most new parents will probably have some knowledge of these nutrients, but here I'll expand on why they are important and how to ensure your baby is getting what she needs. At the end of the chapter, I sum up the nutrient requirements for mom and baby by situation and age.

VITAMIN D: THE SUNSHINE VITAMIN

To give or not to give it to your baby, that's the question. Vitamin D, known as the "sunshine vitamin," has been getting a lot of attention in recent years as research has shown its role in preventing numerous diseases, including multiple sclerosis, type 1 diabetes, and cancer in adults and children. Vitamin D is important for mom during pregnancy as well as breastfeeding to ensure baby has adequate amounts.[11]

Full-term babies are born with vitamin D stores taken from mom that will last for about the first two months of their lives. But premature babies had less time in utero to take vitamin D (and other nutrients) from mom before birth. If you're deficient in vitamin D—perhaps you were pregnant during the winter, you remained inside on bed rest, you're dark-skinned, you wore clothing covering most of your body, or you just weren't in the sun—there will likely have been less to give to your baby. If this is the case, you can improve your baby's levels by supplementing yourself if you're breastfeeding, as vitamin D is one of the nutrients that pass to your baby through breast milk.

Studies show that babies who were exclusively breastfed from birth to six months and have adequate exposure to sunlight (see the box on page 38) are not at risk for developing vitamin D deficiency or rickets.[14] After the first two months as stores start to run out, you'll need to rely on other sources for your baby, including sunlight or UVB rays and breast milk or vitamin D–fortified formula.

> ### Vitamin D: A Hormone and Bone Builder
>
> Vitamin D is not, in fact, a vitamin but a steroid hormone produced by the body after exposure to sunlight.[12] It's stored in the liver, and its role includes promoting the absorption of calcium and phosphorus from the intestines and reabsorption of these bone-building minerals in the kidneys. Deficiency of vitamin D can cause rickets, a bone-softening condition that may lead to fractures and deformities in children. Researchers in Finland also found that children with rickets had an increased risk of type 1 diabetes (juvenile onset).[13]

Vitamin D in breast milk is easily absorbed and acts more effectively than that in formula or foods. It's bound to water-soluble proteins that aid its absorption, which is why it's important for mom to supplement with adequate vitamin D to pass to baby. According to the Public Health Agency of Canada, from July 2002 until December 2003 (18 months), only 69 cases of vitamin D deficiency resulting in rickets were confirmed among children living in Canada.[15] The majority of those cases were infants and toddlers with intermediate and dark skin who had been exclusively breastfed without vitamin D supplementation.

> ### Testing for Vitamin D
>
> If you're concerned about your vitamin D status, ask your doctor for a 25-OH vitamin D blood test. The optimal range is between 32 and 60 nanograms per millilitre (ng/mL).

A Dose of Vitamin D and Safe Sun Exposure

In recent years, the association between exposure to sunlight and cancer has us applying sunscreen liberally on ourselves and our children, limiting the amount of vitamin D our bodies can generate by 95 percent. Sunscreen isn't recommended for babies under six months of age because the absorption of the chemicals found in sunscreen can be harmful. Instead, Health Canada advises that for the first year, babies stay in the shade and wear protective hats, sunglasses, and clothing. Although these recommendations are a safe way to avoid sunburn and other negative effects of UV rays, they can have detrimental effects on vitamin D levels.

Individuals at higher risk of vitamin D deficiency include those who are dark-skinned, wear clothing covering most of the body, use sunscreen daily, live in smoggy cities, or live at higher latitudes, especially in the winter months. In any of these cases, I recommend that a breastfeeding mother supplement her diet with 2000 to 4000 international units (IU) daily. Some of this higher level can be attained from cod-liver oil, which also supplies vitamin A and DHA and is one of the most absorbable sources. Vitamin D supplementation during the summer months may not be as necessary, depending on how much you're out in the sun. If you're outside only on weekends, this may not be quite enough.

A formula-fed baby who's usually covered in the sun should be given a supplement of 400 IU per day. Cod-liver oil is an excellent source of vitamins A and D in a natural ratio that's

Vitamin D Sources

- Sunlight—two hours a week of early morning or late afternoon (before 10 a.m. and after 4 p.m.) sun exposure to the face and hands only. Never risk midday summer sun—your baby's skin will burn if unprotected. Thirty minutes' exposure per week for baby with only a diaper on. Dark-skinned moms and babies will need three to six times more than this. Even in winter, UV rays are around, so your baby will get some benefit from a chilly walk.
- Naturally occurring in foods—fatty fish and fish oils, such as salmon, mackerel, sardines, herring, and cod-liver oil; liver; and egg yolk
- Fortified foods—milk and other dairy products, cereals, margarine, some juices, and alternative milks, such as almond, rice, and soy
- Herb sources—alfalfa and nettle

easy for the body to use: give 1 mL for every 4.5 kg (10 lb) of weight. For example, if you weighed 59 kg (130 lb), you'd need to take 13 mL of cod-liver oil a day, which works out to almost a tablespoon. The oil can also be applied by rubbing it on baby's skin. Otherwise, look for a supplement without flavouring, sugar, or colouring. Carlson makes a product called D

> ### What's the Best Form of Vitamin D?
>
> - Vitamin D3 is the most absorbable form of vitamin D. Margarine and soy products are fortified with D2, a less absorbable form. Read the label of your supplement to ensure it's a D3 source.

Drops that contains nothing artificial and no sugar, and Genestra has an emulsified vitamin D drop. Both are very easy to give to your baby.

Breastfed babies may not need to be supplemented if mom is taking at least 1000 IU vitamin D per day or is out in the sunshine daily. Supplement your baby if he's formula fed, if you're not taking a vitamin D supplement, or if you can't get out in the sunshine every day.

See the Resources at the end of the book for a list of good supplements for mom and baby.

IRON FOR BRAWN, BLOOD, AND BRAINS

Your baby will have stocked up on iron while in utero. This essential mineral supports the development of your baby's brain for cognitive and behavioural maturity and makes hemoglobin, the protein in red blood cells that delivers oxygen to the body's organs, muscles, and tissues.

Iron-deficiency anemia, a lack of adequate red blood cells caused by too little iron, affects about 50 percent of pregnant women. During pregnancy, iron requirements more than double to build new red blood cells in mom and the developing fetus.[16] A blood test will have been done during your pregnancy to check your iron level, and if anemia was found, an iron supplement prescribed. Correcting anemia can take months, and it's important to be retested after a few months to ensure that your levels have improved. Even if you were anemic during pregnancy, one interesting study has shown that your baby won't be predisposed to having low iron stores.[17]

Amazingly, our bodies increase the uptake of iron from foods when our levels are low. Iron is supplied by our diet, and deficiency may be due to numerous reasons: eating too few iron-rich foods, poor absorption of iron, pregnancy, menstruation and heavy periods, long-term blood loss from peptic ulcers, long-term Aspirin use, and certain cancers or malignancies. When supplementing to correct iron deficiency, try to choose a non–ferrous sulfate supplement—either a ferrous gluconate, chelate, or fumarate form. Studies have demonstrated that ferrous sulfate supplements (the most common form of iron, as it's inexpensive) didn't show the expected increase in iron levels. The absorption rate of ferrous sulfate is 10 percent, meaning that if you need to get 10 mg of iron per day, the label of your supplement should read 100 mg of ferrous sulfate. Vitamin C increases the uptake of iron, so take the two together to optimize absorption. Also, take your iron supplement between meals to lessen the chances that other minerals will hinder its absorption.

Iron should only be supplemented after confirming a deficiency. Iron in high doses not only can be toxic, but also competes with other minerals such as calcium, magnesium, and zinc for absorption, possibly leading to deficiencies in these other important minerals.

> ### What Hinders Iron Absorption?
>
> - Calcium and dairy products
> - Black tea and some herb teas (peppermint, camomile)
> - Coffee and cocoa
> - Oxalates found in some dark leafy greens

> ### Signs of Iron Deficiency
>
> Pale skin, fatigue, irritability, dizziness, weakness, shortness of breath, sore tongue, brittle nails, decreased appetite (especially in children), frequent respiratory or intestinal infections, pica (wanting to eat nonfood items such as dirt or ice), headache in the front of your head, itchiness.

YOUR BABY'S BUILT-IN IRON STORE

Healthy, full-term babies have enough iron stores to last for *at least* the first six months of life. Many parents worry that their babies will suddenly run out of their iron stores and become anemic at six months, but current research has shown that they should last from between six and twelve months, perhaps longer in exclusively breastfed babies. So breathe a sigh of relief and don't worry so much while you're still figuring out the introduction of solids or your baby isn't terribly interested in eating.

There appears to be a strong link between low iron levels and birth weight. Preterm babies born with a low birth weight—below 2.5 kg (5.5 lb)—are likely to have low iron. A low-for-gestation birth weight (same as above) or preterm baby would benefit from delayed clamping of the umbilical cord at birth to allow more maternal blood to flow to the baby. Blood drawn from an infant for testing can also contribute to low iron levels.

Your baby is also at risk of iron deficiency during times of rapid weight gain of a month or more (not to be confused with the common growth spurts at three and six weeks, and three and six months, when your baby drinks more than usual). You may see a jump in the weight percentile on your baby's chart, and although this may ease your worry about low weight, it will use up more of baby's already low stores of iron.

If your baby was born at close to her due date at a birth weight above 3 kg (6 lb, 6 oz) and breast- or formula-feeds well, she's unlikely to have low iron. Unless there has been blood loss for some reason, you don't need to be overly nervous about deficiency.

> ### When to Worry about Iron
>
> During the last trimester of pregnancy, your baby nabs iron from your body and begins to store it for future use. This is why preterm babies are at higher risk of low iron levels than babies born at or close to term.

> ### Babies at Increased Risk for Low Iron Levels
>
> - Premature babies, as they take on most of mom's iron during the last trimester.
> - Low birth weight babies less than 3 kg (6 lb, 6 oz).
> - Babies born to mothers with poorly controlled diabetes during pregnancy.
> - Babies fed cow's milk instead of breast milk or formula during the first year.

Avoiding the Side Effects of Iron Supplements

Constipation is the most common side effect of iron supplementation. It may happen during pregnancy when you take your prenatal vitamin (containing iron) or extra iron for diagnosed anemia, or even if you're still taking iron supplements postnatally to correct your iron levels. To decrease constipation, be sure to use the most absorbable forms of iron—ferrous gluconate, chelate, or fumarate. Taking iron between meals with vitamin C increases its absorption, so lower levels may be just as effective. If you're giving iron to your baby—maybe your baby was premature or had blood tests in early infancy—watch for constipation and fussiness as symptoms that he's not tolerating it. If I see this, I recommend ferrum phos tissue salts be given instead. Dosage depends on the individual.

Iron can also be a double-edged sword when it comes to our immune systems. It's important for fighting infection, but at the same time, it's food for bad bacteria such as *E. coli*, *Salmonella*, *Clostridium*, *Bacteroides*, *Escherichia*, and *Staphylococcus*. Because iron in formulas feeds these unfriendly bacteria, it's essential to give infant probiotics to your baby. Read more about formula and iron in Chapter 5.

Iron on Your Plate: Heme and Non-heme Sources

Two types of iron are found in food: heme and non-heme. Heme iron makes up about 40 percent of the iron found in meat, chicken, and fish. The remaining iron in these animal sources as well as all nonmeat foods, including dairy, eggs, fruits, and vegetables, is called non-heme iron. Heme iron is more readily absorbed by the body, at 15 to 35 percent. The amount of non-heme iron that's absorbed varies from 2 to 20 percent or more, depending on the other food and drinks you consume at the same time. You can increase the absorption of non-heme iron in foods by eating them with vitamin C–rich fruits and vegetables and cooking with cast-iron cookware. For example, a bowl of whole grain cereal or toast with almond butter (an iron source) with a glass of orange juice (a vitamin C source) will boost your iron intake. Cooking tomatoes in cast iron especially increases the uptake of iron from the pan due to the tomatoes' acidity.

IRON-RICH FOODS

Meat and Seafood	Beans, Lentils, and Vegetables	Grains and Cereals	Fruit, Juice, and Other
Beef (113 g)* 3.5 mg**	Beans (½ cup/ 125 mL) 2 mg	Pasta (113 g) 1.5 mg	Dried apricots (10 halves) 1.6 mg
Lamb (113 g) 2.5 mg	Chickpeas (½ cup/125 mL) 2 mg	Bagel (28 g) 1 mg	Figs (5) 2 mg
Pork (113 g) 1 mg		Bread (whole wheat, 1 slice) 1 mg	Raisins (113 g) 1.5 mg
Veal (113 g) 1.5 mg	Potato (1 with skin) 2.5 mg	Iron-fortified cereal (28 g) 4–8 mg	Prune juice (227 g) 3 mg
Chicken liver (113 g) 10 mg	Pumpkin (113 g) 1.7 mg	Quinoa flour (½ cup/ 125 mL) 8.5 mg	Nuts (28 g) 1 mg
Beef liver (113 g) 6.5 mg	Peas (113 g) 1 mg	Quinoa, dry (¼ cup/ 50 mL) 3.9 mg	Tofu, firm (85 g) 3.5 mg
Chicken, light meat (113 g) 1 mg	Lentils, cooked (½ cup/125 mg) 3.3 mg	Amaranth (½ cup/ 125 mL) 7.4 mg	Blackstrap molasses (1 tbsp/15 mL) 3.5 mg
Chicken, dark meat, roasted (1 leg and thigh) 2.3 mg	Sweet potatoes (113 g) 1.7 mg	Amaranth flour (½ cup/125 mL) 8.5 mg	Sunflower seeds (2 tbsp/28 g) 1.9 mg
Turkey, light meat (113 g) 1.6 mg	Tomato paste (113 g) 3.9 mg		Pumpkin seeds (2 tbsp/28 g) 4 mg
Turkey, dark meat, roasted (3 slices) 2 mg	Tomato sauce (113 g) 0.8 mg		Infant formula (227 g/8 oz) 3 mg
Clams (113 g) 3 mg			
Oysters (113 g) 8 mg			
Shrimp (113 g) 2 mg			

* Serving size.

** Iron content.

RECOMMENDED DAILY ALLOWANCE (RDA) FOR IRON*
FOR WOMEN AND CHILDREN

Infants from seven to twelve months	11 mg
One to three years old	7 mg
Four to eight years old	10 mg
Pregnant women	27 mg
Breastfeeding mothers	9 mg
Non anemic, non-breastfeeding women	18 mg

Source: Health Canada, "Iron" (June 23, 2009), www.hc-sc.gc.ca/dhp-mps/prodnatur/applications/licen-prod/monograph/mono_iron-fer-eng.php.

* Recommended as an overall daily intake from both food and supplements.

Iron Absorption from Breast Milk, Formula, and Infant Cereal

Iron has its highest absorption rate from breast milk—the vitamin C and high level of lactose in breast milk, as well as the proteins lactoferrin and transferrin, help to increase its absorption.

Iron source and absorbability of iron:

- Breast milk: 50–70 percent
- Iron-fortified dairy formula: 3–12 percent
- Iron-fortified soy formula: 1–7 percent
- Iron-fortified cereal: 4–10 percent
- Cow's milk: 10 percent

Source: Kelly Bonyata, "Is Iron-Supplementation Necessary?" (May 19, 2006), www.kellymom.com/nutrition/vitamins/iron.html.

SUPPLEMENTS FOR EINSTEIN BABY BRAIN

As your baby grows, so does her brain. During the first three months of life, the DHA concentration within your baby's brain will triple, allowing for growth and development of the spinal cord, the neurological system, and, of course, the brain. You will see this growth at each doctor's visit, because along with weight and height, she will measure your baby's head. The increase in head circumference shows that your baby's brain is growing proportionately. DHA makes up 11 percent of the dry weight of the brain, and AA (arachidonic acid), 8 percent, equalling almost 20 percent of its weight. This is a crucial time to ensure that your baby is getting adequate levels of both DHA and AA.

An overwhelming amount of research supports the link between higher intake of DHA and a lower risk of postnatal depression for mom, and an increase in cognitive function and neurological development, lowered risk of hyperactivity and attention deficit disorders, and higher IQ for baby. And did I mention a reduction in severity of allergy? Getting adequate levels of DHA sounds like a no-brainer (sorry, I couldn't resist!).

Of course, we all want smart babies who will one day grow up to be successful in whatever they do. This isn't to say that a child won't reach her full IQ potential without DHA in her diet. But studies do show that breastfed babies who have taken on mom's DHA have, on average, an IQ eight points higher than babies fed formula that wasn't DHA fortified (and, some studies show lower IQ even with fortified formula). This is a significant number. A child who has good concentration and attention span may have an easier time at home, daycare, and school, lessening stress for the whole family, no matter what the age.

AA is also essential for development and works with DHA to enhance its beneficial effects. Formula companies have begun fortifying their products with AA as well as DHA. It's not necessary to supplement with AA, as it's present in our diets worldwide. Arachidonic acid is found in saturated fat, mainly red meat, full-fat dairy products, and fried foods. Most adults typically eat too much of this type of fat. Saturated fat has been linked to an increased risk of cardiovascular disease, including high cholesterol, stroke, and heart attack; Alzheimer's; and other age-related diseases. Our bodies do need a small amount of AA, but not at the levels found in most Western diets. In short, babies need it, but adults, not so much.

Fish Oil DHA

If your baby was born preterm and you're breastfeeding, I recommend that your DHA intake increase to between 2400 mg and 3600 mg per day. Massive brain growth in the third trimester—400 to 500 percent—means that your baby didn't get the chance to finish his brain growth spurt, so you need higher levels of DHA in your cells to pass along through breast milk. Preterm and formula-fed babies should be supplemented with DHA *only* (EPA shouldn't be given to babies under six months of age) at a level of 100 mg per day. DHA-only supplements may be harder to find; see the Resources for recommended brands.

For a full-term baby, you need to take 2400 mg of DHA a day until three months postpartum, at which point you can drop that level down to 1200 mg per day. You can get this amount by taking cod-liver oil or an EPA and DHA supplement (I recommend Genestra's Super DHA Liquid), or by eating fish 24/7. To reach the higher level of DHA from fish, you would need to eat about three pounds of oily fish, such as sardines, mackerel, herring, or wild salmon, *every day*—and more if you eat only white fish. Now I love fish, but I can honestly say there's no way I would be able to eat that amount every day, even if chef Jamie Oliver cooked it for me—not to mention the fact that I'd set the fishmonger up for life financially! And as new moms are notorious for not having as good a diet as they could (they're a bit busy keeping up with the demands of this new life), three pounds of fish daily is probably not on the menu, so either recommendation above is your best option.

As your baby continues to build her brain cell by cell, providing good levels of DHA and AA supports the best possible outcome. I've come across plenty of new moms who were unaware of how crucial these fats are and didn't take their DHA during pregnancy, or with earlier siblings, and are now worried about the implications. Most likely, the baby took these fats from mom during pregnancy and used them for as much brain building as possible. This may lead to a different outcome, but not necessarily a negative one. But of course you want to do your best to help your baby to reach her full potential, so start with a DHA supplement if breastfeeding or give it to your baby or child as soon as possible. Supplementing will still have beneficial effects no matter when you start, even at one year of age.

Your baby needs 100 to 130 mg of DHA daily. DHA is stored in the body, so if you don't give that amount every day, not to worry. But the accumulated level still needs to be reached, even if a supplement isn't given every day. DHA will be present in breast milk if mom is supplementing with it, and some formula companies now fortify their products with DHA and AA. If you're giving your baby DHA/AA-fortified formula, I would recommend only 100 mg of DHA daily on top of what your label quotes. Don't give a baby under six months any supplement containing EPA (a fish oil found in omega-3 or fish oil supplements), as it can compete with absorption of AA.

Unfortunately, I don't have a crystal ball to say what will happen if you don't take your DHA, but after studying nutrition for more than 10 years, I can honestly say that I have only ever seen positive results from taking essential fatty acids in all forms. Now that I specialize in pregnant women, new moms, and their children, not a day goes by that I don't talk about or recommend DHA to mom or baby, and I also take it myself and give it to my children daily (and they love it!).

See the Resources at the end of the book for supplement recommendations.

BUILDING STRONG BONES: IT'S MORE THAN JUST CALCIUM

When your baby is born, he has about 300 bones, some of which are made up of soft, flexible cartilage. As your baby grows, the cartilage is slowly replaced by bone, and the bones grow and fuse together to eventually form 206 adult bones that reach full size by age 25. Your baby accumulated a total of about 30 g of your calcium during pregnancy, mostly during the third trimester, nabbing between 200 and 350 mg a day.[18] That's a huge amount of calcium taken from your stores (oh, what we do for our babies!), but following a calcium-rich diet while breast-feeding should make up for what you lost within a few months after you stop nursing.

Bones store calcium and phosphorus and, in the bone marrow, make blood and immune cells and store fat as an energy source. Bones are made up of a matrix of 25 percent water, 25 percent fibre, and 50 percent mineral salts. Mineral salts of calcium, magnesium, fluoride, and sulfate are deposited between the protein fibres of collagen, crystallize into salts, and make the bone hard. Bones that are too mineralized are brittle and can easily break.

As your baby grows, his bone is destroyed and reformed again and again to eventually reach its full adult shape. Some bone cells eat up the bone, and others rebuild it.

Minerals of calcium, phosphorus, magnesium, boron, and manganese and vitamins D, C, A, and B12 are all used in the complex action of making of bone. Vitamin D increases the absorption of calcium from food but also promotes the removal of calcium from bone. Vitamin C is essential to the collagen matrix—where the calcium is deposited. A deficiency may lead to decreased collagen production, slowing bone growth and delaying healing of broken bones. Vitamin A is involved in breaking down and building up bone, and therefore a deficiency may lead to stunted growth. And, finally, B12 is involved in building up bone after it's broken down. Growth hormone (hGH) is the head honcho when it comes to growth of all tissues, including bone. Too much or little of this hormone can cause over- or undergrowth of bones.

Bones need to be stressed to remain strong. So as your little one grows, walking, running, and jumping are all activities that stress the bone, which in turn keeps the breakdown and buildup of bone in perfect balance.

CALCIUM AND BONES

Despite all the minerals and vitamins that go into building bone, only one usually makes the news—calcium. Calcium is one of the most talked-about minerals and one that I constantly speak about with new moms with regard to when to introduce foods to their babies and toddlers. Dairy products are only one source of calcium; other foods, including nuts and seeds, deliver more calcium than milk (and in a more absorbable form, as they're often raw), with sesame seeds offering 2200 mg of calcium per cup versus 228 mg of calcium per cup of milk. You probably would never eat a cup of sesame seeds at one sitting, but even if you had one-tenth of a cup or one and a half tablespoons, you would get the same amount of calcium as in a cup of milk. Tahini or sesame seed butter is an excellent addition to anyone's diet and is found in hummus, but be careful when introducing it to your baby, as it can be allergenic. Almonds are a powerhouse of calcium, but peanuts offer the least amount of calcium of all nuts and seeds (technically, peanuts are a legume). Salmon and sardines (with bones) rank high in calcium, as do soy, navy beans, blackstrap molasses, amaranth (see page 202 for a yummy recipe), broccoli, and kale. In fact, almost any green leafy vegetable is high in calcium. Milk, however, loses about 50 percent of available calcium in the pasteurization process. Low-fat and skim milk offer even less because the milk fat is used for transportation and absorption of calcium.

Calcium Strippers

So now you know what to eat to get calcium, but on the flip side, what can diminish levels of this mineral? Many factors can contribute to calcium loss in the body:

- High-caffeine coffee, tea, soft drinks, and chocolate increase calcium excretion in the urine.
- Sugar has the same effect as caffeine, and when a food containing calcium and sugar, such as sweetened yogurt, is eaten, the absorption of calcium in the intestines is greatly reduced.[19] Sugar also decreases the amount of phosphorus in the blood.
- High phosphorus intake from meat, grains, and soft drinks can take calcium from bones. Phosphorus and calcium need to be in a particular balance to have a positive effect on bone mineralization. Having too much or too little phosphorus in circulation can have a negative effect on calcium status.
- Salt has the same effect as caffeine and sugar.
- Low vitamin D can lead to low levels of calcium absorption and utilization.
- A high-fibre diet, with most of the fibre coming from wheat, can lead to lowered calcium absorption, as fibre binds to calcium and is excreted from the body.
- Protein eaten in excess depletes calcium substantially in two ways. When protein is eaten, it has an acidic effect on the body, requiring alkaline minerals to buffer the acidity. Calcium, an alkaline mineral, comes out of the bones (along with a few other minerals) to buffer that acid. Junk foods, refined foods, and most cooked foods also have this acid-forming effect on the body. Protein acts as a diuretic, as well, causing the kidneys to send calcium and other minerals out in the urine. This is called a negative calcium balance. In her book *Allergies: Disease in Disguise,* Carolee Bateson-Koch notes that eating too much protein causes more calcium depletion from the bones than consuming too little calcium. Once again, it's all about balance.

A new recommendation to introduce meat at six months as one of the first foods is a concern to me, and the above explains why. A breast- or formula-fed baby is getting the right

> ### Calculating Protein Requirements
>
> To calculate how much protein you or your baby needs, multiply weight in pounds by between .36 to .50 (as an average range, so you aren't number crunching all day) to get the daily protein requirement in grams. Pregnant women need an extra 10 g of protein a day, and lactating moms need an additional 12 g per day.

amount of protein in her diet from her daily milk intake, and my suggestion in Chapters 8 and 9 to delay the introduction of meat also has to do with this calcium balance. Use the calculation in the box below to get a sense of how much protein you and your baby need in a day. There is 0.9 g of protein in 100 mL of breast milk, and as breast milk intake decreases, the protein content increases. It's hard to tell, however, how much a breastfed baby drinks in a day. If you're feeding your baby formula, read the nutritional composition to see how much protein is in it. Similac Advance, for instance, has 1.4 g of protein per 100 mL of formula. Most formulas will have a similar value, as manufacturers must follow guidelines for specific ranges of protein and nutrients.

DAILY CALCIUM REQUIREMENTS

Birth–1 year	400 mg per day
1–3 years	500 mg per day
4–8 years	800 mg per day
Pregnancy, lactation, and adolescence (9–18 years)	1000 mg per day
19–50 years	1300 mg per day
51+ years	1200 mg per day
Individuals at risk for or with osteoporosis	1500 mg per day

Sources: EatRight Ontario, "Calcium Sources," 2009 (www.eatrightontario.ca/en/ViewDocument.aspx?id=203); and Janet Zand, Robert Rountree, and Rachel Walton, *Smart Medicine for a Healthier Child,* 2nd ed. (New York: Penguin Group, 2003).

As we've seen, calcium is important for strong bones, but bone health isn't just about calcium and vitamin D intake. It's also closely related to the hormonal balance of breaking down and building up bone, and to making sure there are limited stressors to calcium. A diet high in protein can be more of a concern, as the body uses calcium to buffer the acidic effect of protein, leading to a negative calcium balance, where what is excreted is more than what is taken in (this also applies to diets high in dairy, wheat, and refined, processed, and packaged food). Food for thought!

PEARLY WHITES: THE START OF HEALTHY BABY TEETH

When your baby is born, her teeth are already hiding in the gums. Well, that's part of the picture. Pediatric dentist Dr. Shonna Masse explains how it all happens:

Your baby is born with teeth already formed in the jaw bone underneath the gums. Baby teeth start to form as early as six weeks in utero, and permanent or adult teeth begin formation as early as five months in utero. The tooth bud goes through many developmental stages and eventually the tooth enamel is calcified, making the hard outer surface of the tooth prior to it erupting through the gums (teething). Calcification of baby teeth begins from about the fourth month in utero, and from birth for permanent teeth. It's busy in that little mouth! Wisdom teeth (third molars) formation starts at about five years of age and usually completes formation by age eight or nine, but may never erupt into the mouth. At each stage of dental development, be it in utero or postpartum, problems can occur which lead to dental abnormalities, such as in the number of teeth (too many or too few), the size or shape of the teeth, the structure of the enamel, the colour, or eruption pattern. It's important to arrange for your child's first dental examination as early as the arrival of their first tooth. This is especially necessary if your child is faced with any dental abnormalities. Your dentist will recommend the appropriate treatment and/or management of the issue.[20]

Good nutrition is essential during pregnancy to support healthy tooth formation. As with bones, minerals of calcium, phosphorus, and vitamins A, C, and D are all used for building teeth. Fluoride is needed in trace amounts to balance mineralization and demineralization when the teeth are exposed to acid. Your baby will have strong teeth before fluoride is introduced in her diet.

Your baby's teeth may tell your dentist a story or two about your pregnancy. Dr. Masse explains, "If something happens during pregnancy, such as some kind of illness, infection, fever, trauma, or use of medication, it may alter the development of the tooth that was forming at that time. It can cause enamel defects that may not be noticed until the tooth erupts." I found that really interesting and wondered what story my first daughter's teeth might have told Dr. Masse, as I broke my wrist when I was five months pregnant with her!

WHAT ARE TEETH MADE OF?

Teeth are made from the same tissue as fingernails, hair, skin, and glands in utero. This tissue then becomes a calcified connective tissue, called *dentin*, which gives the tooth its basic shape and rigidity. Dentin is covered by enamel made up primarily of calcium phosphate and calcium carbonate. Enamel is the hardest substance (as hard as diamonds) in the body, protecting teeth from the constant wear of chewing. It also protects dentin from dissolving in acids that occur in the mouth after eating. The mouth is an alkaline environment with a high pH level, and tooth decay is possible only in the acid environment—at a low pH level. This pH changes after food or drink is ingested.

Dental caries (cavities or tooth decay) happen when bacteria in the mouth act on sugars, found in all carbohydrates, including breast milk, formula, milk, juice, and food, and give off acids that break down or demineralize the enamel. Plaque is formed from bacteria, sugars, and particles that stick to the teeth, covering them and preventing the alkaline saliva from protecting the surface of the teeth from the bacteria. Brushing or rubbing away this plaque from the surface and flossing between tight molars help get rid of plaque, allowing the saliva to once again protect the teeth from bacteria.

DR. DANA COLSON'S TIPS FOR HEALTHY TEETH

- Don't let your baby fall asleep on the breast, as the sugars in breast milk sit in the mouth, and when babies fall asleep, saliva production stops.
- Never allow your baby to go to bed with a bottle of juice, milk, or formula.
- Start brushing teeth from the first eruption. Wipe early teeth with a cloth or gauze, or brush with an appropriately sized toothbrush.
- Floss between back molars if they are close together. If there is sufficient space between the teeth, food will just come out with brushing.

Early Cavity Prevention

"Every time something goes into their mouth, teeth are the tools they're going to use. So thinking early about how to prevent cavities is wise."
—DR. DANA COLSON, DENTIST

THE FIRST DENTIST VISIT

Going to the dentist doesn't have to be a worry. Get your baby or toddler used to going to the dentist by taking him with you when you go. Let him see what it's all about and how mommy or daddy does it, or let older siblings show younger ones how it's done. Find a pediatric or general dentist, who should have all sorts of kid-friendly names for the tools they use. One of my favourites is "Mr. Thirsty," who sucks out the saliva in the mouth. Some dentists recommend a first visit at about age three, and pediatric dentists like to see the little teeth as they come in, so by age one. After taking my daughters to the dentist regularly, I understand why some dentists recommend a slightly older first visit—often children are scared or shy when someone they don't know looks in their mouth. At the same time, good oral health and cavity prevention start early, so the more you know as the teeth erupt, the better equipped you'll be.

When you visit the dentist and either you or your child needs a filling or sealants to cover the teeth, ask questions and do your homework before you go ahead. If X-rays are needed, see if your dentist does digital X-rays, which give off 90 percent less radiation. Ask about the composite used to fill or seal teeth and any harmful chemicals it may contain. Dentists commonly suggest sealing teeth, especially those with deep grooves in them. While there has been a movement away from amalgam or mercury fillings because of the known negative neurotoxin effects, the newer white or composite fillings may contain bisphenol A (BpA), a chemical also known for its potentially harmful effects on the nervous system, as well as its link to cancer and other health issues. Remember this if you need any dental work while breastfeeding, as the toxins may get into your breast milk and thus into your baby at a crucial time of development.

THUMB SUCKING AND SOOTHERS

Some parents worry about thumb sucking because a thumb isn't as easy to take away as a soother or pacifier. For some babies, self-soothing with fingers or thumb is comforting, and that's something that shouldn't be discouraged. I recall my second daughter sucking her fingers as a newborn, and it was a beautiful thing when she soothed herself back to sleep on many occasions (although that habit didn't last long!).

Dentists don't seem too worried about the use of the thumb or soother, up until the age of three, anyway. In my interview with her, Dr. Colson said that she's not opposed to either, as both help develop the open airway that's so important for good sleep. Use an orthodontic soother, which lessens the likelihood of changing the angle of the upper teeth.

Have you ever put your baby's soother in your mouth after it dropped on the floor to "clean" it? This practice is of concern to pediatric dentist Dr. Shonna Masse. She explains, "Oral bacteria can be spread between parent and child. It may be done by something as innocent as sharing a utensil or a kiss, but the bacteria are microscopic and transfer easily. If there is an infection or cavity-causing bacteria in mom or dad's mouth, then it can be shared with the baby and may lead to oral health issues, namely cavities for the child."[21] So hang on to the soother until you can wash it somewhere other than your mouth!

TRICKY TEETHING

Teething is painful for everyone involved. Your baby is unhappy while you try to figure out what you can do to help her weather the erupting tooth. Teething can happen without a tooth making an appearance *for months*. Your baby might showing signs of drooling, fussiness, chewing on anything and everything, low-grade fever, pulling on her ears, diarrhea or constipation, lack of appetite for food, bum rash usually close to the anus, and red cheeks for months before a tooth breaks through the gums.

Babies can start teething at a young age, when you probably wouldn't attribute any of the above symptoms to teething. Your baby may sail through the first tooth but have more symptoms with the next one. Signs of teething come and go and can be worse at night, followed by long days of clinginess and irritability. Your baby may want to nurse more for comfort, chew at your knuckles, and be held all day long.

Your mission is to try to help your baby, and yourself, through these teething episodes. Dampen a clean baby facecloth with water and put it in the freezer, offer a hard toy to chew on or a large, cold whole carrot (so it won't break off and become a choking hazard) or even an ice cube wrapped in a cloth to numb the teeth. A common misconception is that teething biscuits help babies with teething. Not only do they *not* help, but they're often full of ingredients that baby hasn't tried yet; they might contain wheat flour and sugar, which suppress the immune system at a time when baby's more susceptible to sickness; and I've even seen one product sweetened with honey, which is on the avoid list for babies under one year. And when your baby is teething he usually loses his appetite for solid foods, but not usually his "milk."

Symptoms of diarrhea are more common than constipation, but bowel movements can change either way depending on your baby. Her stool and urine can become more acidic, leading to red bum cheeks and soreness that sometimes can be raw and bleed. A protective barrier cream, especially a natural one, is perfect for this kind of rash. I have also seen eczema flare up with teething episodes in some babies.

Is It a Cold or a New Tooth?

It's easy to confuse teething with the start of a cold, as symptoms can sometimes seem similar: runny nose, low-grade fever (under 38°C/100°F), ear pulling, and fussiness. When teeth are starting to erupt, the immune system can get confused and see the teeth as a foreign invader breaking through the skin, and send out the immune army to deal with it. While the immune system's busy, your baby may be prone to colds, infections, and flare-ups of eczema. Support his little body with immune-boosting probiotics, homeopathic teething remedies, and lots of comfort.

Homeopathy, a safe, alternative medicine based on treating the symptoms of ailments, offers various remedies that can make a world of difference for your baby's teething symptoms, and you often see fast results. Consult a homeopath or naturopath to match your list of teething symptoms to particular remedies. Medication is often a last resort to help everyone sleep for more than an hour or two, and sometimes parents will use teething gels. But be careful with teething gels (other than homeopathic ones), as they can numb not only the gums but also the tongue and lips. Be sure to read the label carefully when giving any medication to your baby, and consult the pharmacist if you have questions.

BRUSHING AWAY THE BUGS

Start brushing your baby's teeth as soon as they erupt with a cloth or piece of gauze wrapped around your finger. As the teeth continue to erupt, it becomes more important to wipe or brush them daily. Once the premolars come in at around one year, and then molars at about two years, those bite surfaces need to be brushed well to remove any debris. And don't forget in between those teeth too—a common area for plaque to build and bacteria to live.

The three dentists I spoke with before writing this section all agreed that toothpaste isn't necessary for your baby, and two of them said that you never need to use it. Toothpaste can be something sweet to entice your baby or toddler to brush, but it isn't really necessary (they usually just suck it off, anyway). If you do want to use toothpaste, find one that is fluoride free and read the ingredients. Most toothpastes, even those sold in health food stores, contain sodium lauryl sulphate, a chemical foaming agent also used in skin care and bath products. And if you don't want to offer blue bubble gum–flavoured toothpaste, look anywhere other than the pharmacy. Search for safe products on the Skin Deep website (www.cosmeticsdatabase.com). All dentists recommend avoiding fluoride tooth-paste until about age three or until your child is able to spit out the toothpaste during brushing, as ingesting fluoride is not recommended.

Juice versus Water

Giving juice at bedtime is a definite no-no, but even offering juice throughout the day can leave the sugars hanging around in crevices and in between the teeth. As Dr. Robert Penning explains, "As a dentist, I tell parents that after milk and water, most other beverages are largely entertainment. Much of the decay I see would likely disappear if other beverages were eliminated."[22] If you do give juice, which I don't recommend until after two years of age, dilute it with water and give with a meal or in one sitting rather than all day long.

To sum up the nutritional nuts and bolts you and your baby need, here's a handy reference chart.

SUMMARY OF SUPPLEMENTS FOR MOM AND BABY

	Vitamin D*	Iron	DHA*	Calcium/ Magnesium	Probiotic
Pregnant woman	1000 IU or sun exposure daily	27 mg	1200 mg first and second trimesters, and 2400 mg from third trimester	1300 mg/ 600–800 mg	18 billion *L. acidophilus* and 6 billion *Bifidobacterium* once to twice daily***
Breastfeeding mom	2000–4000 IU or more than two hours of sun a week	9 mg	2400 mg until baby is three months old, then 1200 mg per day	1300 mg/ 600–800 mg	6 billion *L. acidophilus* and 2 billion *Bifidobacterium* once to twice daily***
Non-breastfeeding mom	1000 IU	18 mg	600 mg	800 mg/ 400 mg	6 billion *L. acidophilus* and 2 billion *Bifidobacterium* once to twice daily***
Preterm baby	400 IU	2–4 mg/ kg/day**	2400 mg–3600 mg taken by mom while breastfeeding or 100 mg of DHA only for baby	Not generally supplemented	1 billion *L. acidophilus*, 1 billion *L. casei*, and 1 billion *Bifidobacterium infantis* once to twice daily***
Breastfed full-term baby	None if mom is supplementing, or 400 IU if not	None	None if mom is taking the above	400 mg/ 200 mg	1 billion *L. acidophilus*, 1 billion *L. casei*, and 1 billion *Bifidobacterium infantis* once to twice daily***
Formula-fed full-term baby	400 IU if not exposed to sunlight	None	100 mg	400 mg/ 200 mg	1 billion *L. acidophilus*, 1 billion *L. casei*, and 1 billion *Bifidobacterium infantis* once to twice daily***

* Vitamin D and DHA can also be obtained from cod-liver oil while breastfeeding only. Not suitable during pregnancy. Use 1 mL (1/4 tsp) for every 4.5 kg (10 lb) of weight. For example, if you weighed 130 lb (59 kg), you would need to take 13 mL of cod-liver oil a day, which works out to almost a tablespoon.

** Should be prescribed by doctor.

*** Preferably a human or human microflora (HMF) strain

4

THE WHITE STUFF
Breastfeeding

Breast milk or formula is your baby's main source of nutrition for the first year of life, and it's her *only* source of nutrition for the first six months before she starts on solids. When you think back to your newborn, and the huge gains in weight, height, head circumference, and progression of development she's made over the first six months, it's amazing that just the white stuff (I know it's not really white, but it's catchy) has provided all the nourishment for this remarkable growth.

Whether to breastfeed your baby or not is often a hot topic before you give birth, and, as usual, everyone has their own advice and experience to offer—good and bad. If you took prenatal classes, you might have talked about breastfeeding or watched a video that showed you how to get baby's tiny mouth to open wide enough to take the whole nipple. But nothing really prepares you for the actual experience.

For some, the thought of breastfeeding is foreign, and the decision to breastfeed or not is a real struggle. Unfortunately, it's not for everyone. Others decide that they are going to breastfeed exclusively and are devastated when it doesn't work out. Feeding your baby may not go as smoothly as you'd hoped for a multitude of reasons, whether you are breast- or formula-feeding. But I've heard some wonderful success stories from new moms who, with great determination and excellent support, worked through the challenges of breastfeeding.

In my own early days of nursing, I had different challenges with the latch. I found that both my daughters reacted to foods I had eaten—dairy, wheat, sugar, and chocolate were the worst. Although I practise what I preach most of the time and follow a healthy diet, I'm not a saint, and every now and then I would sit and indulge in some of my favourite Stilton cheese or focaccia dunked in extra-virgin olive oil and balsamic vinegar, or need sugary chocolate to keep going. Every time I ate something I wasn't supposed to, a rash, constipation, or discomfort would show up in my babies within the next day or two. I felt like the worst mother in the world for being so weak as to eat something that I knew might cause a reaction. But although we all try to do the best we can for our children, we are still human.

SUPER-POWERED BREAST MILK: THE BENEFITS OF BREASTFEEDING

Anyone who thinks that breastfeeding is the most "natural" thing for a new mom to do is only partly right. Breastfeeding does not come naturally or easily to every new mom. Yet everywhere you turn, you're told that breast is best. Well it is, but it also may be more challenging than you thought.

Breastfeeding is a new skill that both you and your baby need to learn. Even if this is your second baby, you might need a bit of practice to get it right. If you're having difficulty, it's crucial that you seek help from a lactation consultant, breastfeeding clinic, or your midwife (see the Resources section for suggestions).

Mastering the latch of your baby's mouth to your nipple can be a challenge. But once your baby does latch on, he'll receive the appropriate amount of colostrum (the first fluid delivered to your newborn) or milk. A poor latch can lead to your baby having insufficient nutrition; dehydration; inefficient clearing of bilirubin, leading to prolonged jaundice; or a lack of bowel movements, including meconium (the first, tarlike poo), and urination. In mom, an improper latch can cause low milk production from a lack of nipple stimulation and sore or cracked nipples while nursing. These are the many reasons why it's essential to master a good latch as quickly as you can, and to get help when you need it.

Breast milk is the perfect food—the gold standard—for your baby. It makes complete sense that human milk is the best milk for its offspring. An exceptional amount of research has gone into the lifelong benefits of breastfeeding for both

Sweeping Statements

I was told that losing half my nipple to breastfeeding my first child was nothing to be concerned about—many women continue to breastfeed through worse circumstances; just press on, it's bound to get better. Yeah, right!
—CATHY, MOM OF THREE

mom and baby. One study reported that women who breastfed for one year or more over their lifetime were less likely to develop high blood pressure, diabetes, high cholesterol, breast cancer, or cardiovascular disease than women who never nursed.[23] Scientists have studied breast milk for years to try to uncover every aspect of what it does, how it does it, and why. I'll share as many of its benefits as I can here, so you'll find out more than just a few well-known facts.

IMMUNITY

Breast milk provides antibodies for your baby to protect her body from foreign invaders until her immune system has matured. Colostrum, the first milk your baby receives after birth, is loaded with secretory immunoglobulin A, or sIgA (see Chapter 7 for more details). This antibody guards the mucosal entranceways to the body—the nose, eyes, mouth, and, most importantly, digestive system—by binding to bacteria and viruses and quashing them. Amazingly, sIgA is found in higher levels in the milk of mothers of preterm babies, who, with their premature immune systems, are even more susceptible to bacteria and viruses.[24] Babies who are born vaginally take on good bacteria, *Lactobacillus* and *Bifidobacterium*, from the birth canal, as well as not-so-good bacteria that live around the anal area of the digestive tract. I know it's not a nice thought, but this is a crucial step for stimulating the newborn immune army to start working toward balancing itself. Your skin also offers good and bad bacteria to your baby's digestive system through his mouth, from the first skin-to-skin contact and breastfeed. You provide your own sIgA to your baby through colostrum and breast milk, giving your baby a head start in protecting himself from the bad bacteria you share with him.[25] Also, sIgA allows for the colonization of friendly bacteria, *Lactobacillus acidophilus* and *Bifidobacterium,* in the intestines without mounting an attack—another key aspect of developing a strong immune system.

Breastfeeding increases the size of baby's thymus, a gland in the immune army.[26] The thymus is where immune cells, called T-cells, including killer T-cells, mature before heading out into the battlefield of the body. The larger the thymus, the more T-cells are produced, and the stronger the immune army. The more your baby breastfeeds, the larger the size of the thymus.

VITAMINS AND MINERALS

Breast milk contains the most absorbable forms of all vitamins and minerals, especially iron and zinc. Although iron concentrations are low in breast milk, it provides maximum absorption.

Zinc blood levels are higher in breastfed babies than formula-fed babies, even though the concentration level of zinc is higher in formula milk.[27] Once again, it all comes down to absorbability. Water-soluble vitamins (B vitamins and vitamin C) are taken from mom's diet and passed on to baby. Fat-soluble vitamins A and E are found in the hind milk, or fatty milk, in perfect proportions and are taken from your stores, rather than from your diet or supplements.[28] Vitamins are directed to the mammary glands, away from use by your own body[29]—all more reason to take your pre- and postnatal vitamins and eat a nutrient-rich diet.

NOURISHMENT

Breast milk has the right proportions of carbohydrate, fat, and protein for your baby's growth and development. Here's a look into the specific components of breast milk, in some detail and with a bit of science, as it's fascinating to see what it's made up of.

Fats

Essential fatty acids DHA and AA are found in abundance in breast milk. They are extremely important for the development of the brain, retina, and neurological system and may even help decrease the potential for allergies. Mom doesn't need to supplement with AA—the diet easily supplies what her baby needs.

DHA, on the other hand, is needed in such large quantities that mom usually needs to supplement with fish oils containing DHA. Hind milk has twice the level of fat than fore milk (the first, carbohydrate-rich milk your baby gets).[30] Breast milk contains not only these two fats, but also a host of other lesser-known essentials, including lauric, myristic, palmitic, stearic, oleic, linoleic, and linolenic acids.[31] In a clever twist, breast milk also contains lipase, a fat-digesting enzyme that's essential to the digestion of these important fats because a newborn baby's digestive system isn't mature enough to produce its own enzymes.[32] Lipase then stays in the digestive tract, furthering the digestion of all fats found in breast milk.

Protein

Whey and casein are the main proteins found in breast milk. The immune protein sIgA and binding proteins lactoferrin, folate, and cobalamine (B12) are also components of breast milk and help with baby's absorption of iron, folic acid, and B12.[33] Lactoferrin has many other important functions, such as providing antiviral effects against fungus such as *Candida albicans,* lowering the risk of urinary tract infections, promoting the growth of *Bifidobacteria* in the digestive tract, and helping the growth of the mucosal lining of the intestines.[34]

Carbohydrates

Lactose is the primary carbohydrate that gives your baby energy for every bodily process. It also enhances the absorption of calcium, iron, magnesium, and manganese.[35]

The largest solid component in human milk is oligosaccharides. These carbohydrates are fuel for the beneficial bacteria in the digestive tract. They also take up residence in the walls of the intestines, where, like posters put up on a wall, they cover as much space as possible so that other pathogens or bad guys can't move in and cause an infection or illness.

Water makes up 87.5 percent of breast milk.[36] Hint, hint—how much water have you drunk today? My midwife always told me to drink a glass of water every time I breastfed. This was great advice—all I had to do was remember to pour the glass before I sat down to nurse!

LOWERED RISK OF OBESITY

An appetite-regulating hormone called leptin is found in breast milk.[37] This hormone also stimulates the immune army and its hard-working soldiers. (I talk more about the immune army in Chapter 7.) The presence of this hormone may be the reason for the decreased incidence of obesity in breastfed babies.

GROWTH

Breast milk contains nucleotides that cow's milk does not. Nucleotides are the building blocks needed by DNA and RNA to support the growth and development of all systems in the body, including the immune system.[38]

Healthy Mouth

Breastfeeding encourages healthy muscle development through the suckling action of the jaw and mouth. However, for healthy teeth, dentist Dr. Dana Colson suggests, "Try not to let your baby fall asleep on the breast, as the sugars in the breast milk sit in the mouth and when baby falls asleep, saliva production stops. Saliva protects the teeth from the acidity of the sugars." Good advice, although sometimes easier said than done.

MAKING THE GOOD STUFF BETTER: WHAT CAN YOU DO?

If you're a nursing mom, you'll need a good-quality daily pre- or postnatal multi-nutrient. Although not all the vitamins and minerals in a multi will be passed on

---

Sweeping Statements

My daughter got an eye infection, and I was told to dab breast milk on her eye to clear it up. Breast milk also was suggested to heal cracked nipples and diaper rash. It worked, but I was skeptical at first! (Express a bit into a cup and use a dropper to apply to any area.)
—LEAH, MOM OF ONE

to your baby, it covers the extra demands on your own nutrient stores. Supplements in capsule form have far better absorption than hard tablets. The labels of some better-quality multivitamins might suggest taking two to four per day. They just can't fit all those nutrients into one capsule!

Your dietary or supplemental iron intake does not seem to have a direct influence on the level of iron in breast milk. Ensuring that you're not iron deficient is important for your well-being, but breast milk uses the iron stored in your body to nourish your baby.[39]

Vitamin D levels can be increased with supplementation and sun exposure. It might take about two weeks to influence the level of vitamin D in breast milk, but it can increase dramatically while providing the appropriate amounts to your baby, whatever level you are exposed to or taking orally.[40]

Water-soluble vitamins, including the B family of vitamins (B1, B2, B3, B5, B6, folic acid, and B12) and vitamin C are found to increase in breast milk when present in mom's diet, either from food or supplements. Vegan and some vegetarian mothers are more at risk for vitamin B12 deficiency because B12 is found in eggs, fish, dairy, and meat. If you're deficient, your baby can be as well, so if you're following a vegan diet, be sure to supplement with adequate B12. A word of caution with B6: Taking more than what's found in your multi may cause a decrease in breast milk production.

Although the probiotics *Bifidobacterium* and *Lactobacillus acidophilus* can't get into the breast milk directly, as they live in the digestive tract and don't reach the bloodstream, they do enhance certain immune components in your body. Those components then pass into the breast milk from your bloodstream, having a positive immune-enhancing effect in your baby.

Begin Probiotics at Birth

I highly recommend giving your baby her own supplement of *Bifidobacterium infantis* and *Lactobacillus acidophilus* starting at birth. These friendly bacteria have been well studied for their benefits, which reach well into adulthood, including reducing the potential for allergies, and they show no adverse affects.[41] I recommend giving at least three billion live cultures (or total bacteria) from human strains daily after nursing. A powder form is easily given off your finger or sprinkled on your nipple (a bit more hit-and-miss). See Resources for brand suggestions and page 57 for specific strains.

The essential fatty acids DHA and AA are taken from your body, either from red blood cells or tissues such as the brain (remember mommy brain?), to support the development of your baby's brain, retina, and neurological system. Taking 2400 mg of DHA in the last trimester and for the first three months of your baby's life has far-reaching benefits, including a much

> ### Vegetarian and Vegan Moms
>
> Vegetarian and vegan moms have 50 to 70 percent less DHA in their breast milk than fish-eating moms.[42] An algae source DHA supplement is essential for those who don't eat fish (see Resources for brand suggestions).

lower risk of postpartum depression and increased IQ and development in your baby (see the table on page 57 for a list of which supplements to take, and when). Saturated or unhealthy trans fats that you eat also make it into breast milk, so it's advisable to avoid fried foods, red meat, and prepackaged fatty foods as much as possible, since these fats are associated with cardiovascular disease.

As we've seen, many elements of what you ingest reach your baby. This also applies to medication. Before taking any medication, contact www.motherisk.org or refer to *Dr. Jack Newman's Guide to Breastfeeding*.

> ### Sweeping Statements
>
> Breastfeeding myth: I was told that I needed to drink milk and eat butter so that I could provide breast milk!
> —SHAIROSE, MOM OF ONE

BREASTFEEDING CHALLENGES

As mentioned earlier, breastfeeding is not without its difficulties. These can include serious situations of pain or infections in mom. Here's what can happen and how to avoid it.

BLOCKED DUCTS

Blocked ducts can happen at any stage of breastfeeding. They're most common in women with adequate milk supply but inadequate breast drainage during feeds. This can lead to milk stasis, or clogging of milk in the ducts, resulting in painful, localized swelling around the affected duct that's sometimes visible as a tiny white plug on the nipple or a palpable, tender lump.[43] Nursing with your baby's chin pointed *toward or in line with* the blocked duct aids in releasing the blockage. The strength of sucking is more powerful from the lower jaw than the upper jaw, so try new positions to pull that blockage through while compressing your breast with your hand to drain it toward the nipple (for visual help, visit the Newman Breastfeeding Clinic and Institute website at www.ncbi.ca).

CRACKED NIPPLES

Most nursing moms will end up with cracked nipples, caused by their stretching as baby draws the breast tissue into her mouth. Cracked nipples can happen because of an incorrect latch when the baby doesn't take enough of the areola into the mouth and mainly sucks on the nipple. Correcting the latch with support from a lactation consultant or by making sure that you get the whole of the areola into your baby's mouth, with the bottom lip visibly curled away from the breast, should ease this often excruciating condition, which can lead to bleeding or infection. Natalie Rogers, a child birth educator who specializes in lactation and holistic nutrition, suggests, "When cracks appear, a frequent recommendation is to rub a little expressed breast milk onto the nipple after each feed (breast milk has antibacterial and healing properties!), and the application of aloe gel, lanolin, calendula ointment and/or olive oil are all thought to be healing for cracks."[44] You can try a nipple shield temporarily to let the cracks heal, then go back to nursing without it. I was given a tincture with St. John's wort and calendula to dilute and drizzle on my cracked nipples, and it healed them right away. Consult a herbalist for the right product, or see the resource section for what I used.

MASTITIS

Mastitis is a bacterial infection of the breast. The first symptoms are tiredness, localized breast tenderness, and a flu-like muscular aching, followed by fever and swelling and redness of the affected breast. Factors contributing to mastitis include plugged ducts, stress, fatigue, cracked or fissured nipples, bra constriction, engorgement or milk stasis, and an abrupt change in frequency of feedings.[45] Mastitis can happen at any stage of breastfeeding. Treatment usually includes frequent nursing of affected breast, application of moist heat (such as a hot face cloth or shower), increased fluids, bed rest, and antibiotics if the infection does not resolve within two to four days. If you do take antibiotics, remember to follow up with probiotics, both for yourself and for baby, during and after the treatment, as it can lead to candida or thrush.

I had mastitis only once, thank goodness, when my second daughter was 10 months old. It came out of the blue, and I was surprised to have such painful symptoms at that stage of breastfeeding. I contacted my naturopath, who asked detailed questions about my symptoms and prescribed a homeopathic remedy of belladonna (for heat and redness) that cleared it up within 24 hours. I also increased my garlic intake and took higher levels of vitamin C and probiotics to support my immune system. It's helpful to have a naturopath or homeopath to call on in times like this. Homeopathy can have amazing results when you take the right remedy for your symptoms. See the resource section for suggestions of how to find a naturopath or homeopath in your area, or ask friends as word-of-mouth referrals are often best.

YEAST, THRUSH, OR CANDIDA INFECTIONS

I've talked many times about good bacteria and bad bacteria. Well, this is one of the bad guys. Classed as a fungus, *Candida albicans* is present in all of us, but the problem arises when we have higher levels in the digestive tract, usually after a course of antibiotics. According to *Dr. Jack Newman's Guide to Breastfeeding*, the shooting or burning pain of thrush can begin late in the feeding or afterward, it's usually worse in the evenings, and it's felt throughout the breast and sometimes in mom's shoulder or back, lasting for minutes or hours and starting at any age of the baby. A common first treatment of thrush is a purple liquid called Gentian

From the Mouths of Moms

Within a week of giving birth to my son, I had a full-blown case of mastitis. I was put on antibiotics, which caused the flare-up of candida symptoms. Looking for help, I first worked with my naturopath to help rid my body of the candida that had reappeared numerous times throughout my life and was back again. I also visited a number of breastfeeding clinics in and around Toronto, trying to get relief from the three subsequent bouts of mastitis that occurred within the first two months of my son's life. I believed the mastitis might also be occurring because of Owen's latch, so I ventured to Jack Newman's renowned breastfeeding clinic, only to be told that his latch was fine and he seemed to be guzzling quite well.

Owen cried a lot in those early days. We thought he was colicky, and his dad would take him for drives in the middle of most nights, hoping to lull him back to sleep. A friend suggested at the one-and-a-half-month mark that Owen might be hungry, and perhaps all my issues with mastitis had reduced my breast milk. The thought hadn't crossed my mind, as Owen was gaining weight and meeting all his milestones. She showed me how to supplement Owen's intake by tube feeding with formula, and his crying miraculously stopped. To stimulate my milk production, I started a cocktail of milk thistle and fenugreek, but nothing seemed to work until I was introduced to John Redden, a medical herbalist in Toronto. After hearing my story, he recommended his herbal "galactagogue" called Lactaid, a natural product made from herbs such as borage, goat's rue, and fennel. Within two days, I had all the breast milk I needed and more. I joyfully threw away all the tubes, bottles, and formula I'd used to supplement my breast milk, and for the first time, felt the elation in being able to successfully feed my son with my own milk.
—CAROLYN, MOM OF OWEN

Violet, which is applied around the nipple and areola and in the baby's mouth on a Q-tip. Antifungal medications are often prescribed; Dr. Newman recommends grapefruit seed extract. I've seen homeopathic remedies provide fast and safe help for both mom and baby. Giving probiotics to both mom and baby in higher doses is imperative.

BABY'S REACTIONS TO BREAST MILK

Some of the foods or drinks you consume may not agree with your baby. Common symptoms include gassiness, fussiness, diarrhea, constipation, rashes, runny nose, and spitting up. I've seen remarkable improvement in babies when mom removes certain foods from her diet.

I recall a mom in one of my Mommy Chef cooking classes who cut dairy out of her diet to help her son's skin rash. This cleared up the rash, and to her amazement he stopped spitting up. She had no idea that her dairy intake could affect him—her doctor had told her that some babies are just "spitter-uppers" and to just live with it.

Common foods that may upset your baby are dairy products, including milk (usually the worst), cheese, yogurt, and cottage cheese; chocolate (sorry); caffeine (again, sorry); melons, cucumbers, peppers, citrus fruits and juices, and spicy foods. Gas-forming foods can also be a contributing factor, such as cauliflower, broccoli, brussels sprouts, cucumbers, red and green peppers, onions, beans, and legumes. These are the most likely culprits, but not all of them may affect your baby.

A milk allergy in your baby may show; although he's not yet drinking cow's milk, the reaction may come from *your* dairy intake. This allergy often presents itself as discomfort such as gassiness, colic-like symptoms, and pulling up of the legs while crying; skin reactions such as eczema; or, even worse, blood in the stool. Most doctors will suggest taking dairy out of your diet in the case of bloody stool. Soy should come out of the diet as well. Both are highly allergenic foods.

This may seem like a very limited diet, but look at what you're eating in the largest quantities. Often it's wheat and dairy. There are many alternatives to these foods, so you won't go hungry, and I wouldn't suggest restricting your diet too much as you need nutrients and calories for your body and breast milk production. With the help of a nutritionist, you can eat a super-healthy diet without the foods that are upsetting your baby.

Start by keeping a food diary and writing down your baby's reactions next to the foods you've eaten to see what might be a trigger. Remember, though, that it may take some time for the food you've just eaten to get into your breast milk and be digested by your baby, so with any reaction you'll need to look back a meal or two, and maybe even at what you ate yesterday. Next, eliminate any suspected foods to see if this has a positive effect on your baby. Think about whatever you eat or drink every day and more than once a day and see if taking it out of your diet for at least two weeks helps. Food intolerance tests also can be done to see what you or your baby is reacting to (see Chapter 7).

After my first daughter ended up with a scarlet-red bum rash when she started on solids, I consulted a naturopath, who agreed that something I was eating was leading to her yeast symptoms (the type of red bum rash was indicative of yeast). She sent us for food-sensitivity testing. We were both tested with the adult food list of about 300 foods (the testing is noninvasive, by the way). My results showed my own sensitivities, and my daughter's list showed some of the same sensitivities and more! I now had two lists to follow. Out went gluten, dairy, sugar, some fruits, and even goat's milk products. I followed a very limited diet for a few months, and then we went for retesting. Slowly, my daughter's "safe foods" list expanded as her skin problems cleared up. She stopped breastfeeding at around 20 months, and I continued to have her tested to see how her body changed as she got older. When she was three years old, gluten (which includes wheat) was finally on the "OK" list, but sugar and dairy never made it off the "avoid" list.

BREAST MILK APLENTY

Breast milk production is all about supply and demand. A good latch in the early days, especially in the first hours of baby's life, ensures that prolactin, the hormone that produces breast milk, is stimulated to keep it flowing. Support is essential to get that latch just right so that you don't suffer nipple pain, cracking, or infection.

Many mothers have told me that they began formula-feeding because of a lack of breast milk—or because they thought they weren't producing enough milk. But before giving up on nursing, I would suggest consulting with an expert such as a lactation consultant to uncover the reasons behind low milk supply and to confirm that there is, in fact, an issue here. Softer breasts might make you think that you aren't producing as much milk, but your body has regulated its production and your breasts aren't as full as in the early days. Make an appointment with a breastfeeding clinic or lactation consultant as early as you can, even before the birth, just to make sure you're on the right track, and learn how to

Getting the Milk Flowing

Low breast milk production is almost always tied to poor technique and insufficient nipple stimulation. The more nipple stimulation there is, the more the hormone prolactin is produced, and the more milk the breast makes. But if mom isn't latching baby properly or leaving him on long enough to drain the breast, her body will start to slow down production. Very young babies will need to be awakened if they fall asleep at the breast, especially if they have come through a medicated labour and delivery (epidurals make them sleepy). It's not always understood that babies need to feed often to build up mom's milk supply in the first few days. There is an optimum time for mom to get baby to the breast after birth, within the first half an hour to hour after birth, to set up the hormones that ensure adequate milk supply. That's not to say that you can't build up a good milk supply if you can't breastfeed right away, but it is an added advantage.

Nighttime is the optimum time for baby to have unrestricted access to the breast. Weaning baby off night feeds too early can result in reduced milk production because prolactin levels are higher at night. Stress is a big factor when it comes to having enough milk for a baby. Mom's inability to relax interferes with the "let-down" reflex while nursing and affects how much milk the baby gets. Physiological issues that can affect milk supply are breast surgery where milk ducts have been severed or removed, or an actual deficit in breast glandular tissue, which is very rare. Other than that, it's pretty much technique and frequency.

—NATALIE ROGERS, CBDE RHN (CHILDBIRTH EDUCATOR)

improve the latch or hold. Some medications, such as estrogen in birth control pills, may reduce milk production, and fertility hormones, if you're working on baby number two or three, may also decrease supply. Breast augmentation and especially breast reduction might lead to lower production. In his *Guide to Breastfeeding,* Dr. Jack Newman notes, "There is no doubt that some women are unable to produce enough milk, just as some people do not produce enough insulin or thyroid hormone. But this does not mean that these mothers cannot, or should not breast feed."[46] Dr. Newman supports the use of a lactation aid to keep milk production going, as well as still trying to feed from the breast. He's of the opinion that if you're producing less breast milk than your baby requires, some is better than none, and you shouldn't stop. He opposes giving formula in the first 24 hours of a baby's life, as it can be detrimental to mom's milk supply and baby loses out on colostrum.

Try these tips to increase your milk supply:

- Make sure you're getting enough calories in your diet. While breastfeeding, you need to eat an additional 500 calories—for example, one cup of Mom's Super-Powered Smoothie (see the recipe on page 35). Dieting is not advised, as your breast milk may decrease with a lower calorie intake. Dieting also liberates stored toxins and waste products that can get into your breast milk. I highly recommend seeing a nutritionist, who can help you deal with your weight challenges while maintaining a healthy diet for you and baby. See the list of foods to eat every day (pages 33–35), "Healthy Super-Snacks" (page 7), and "Mommy Meals" (page 32). Breastfeeding actually speeds up weight loss without a calorie-restricted diet. Sounds much better than running on a treadmill, doesn't it?
- Drink enough water. Dehydration will zap your energy and is detrimental to overall health, so aim to drink 2 to 3 L of water per day. Your body needs water to make breast milk, and preference goes to the baby, as usual, so you might suffer from low energy, dry skin, or constipation as a result of not drinking enough water.
- Check how much vitamin B6 you are taking. The level in your multinutrient should be fine, but too much B6 can reduce breast milk production. Avoid taking extra B6, such as in a B complex supplement.
- Try the herbs fenugreek and blessed thistle. Dr. Jack Newman recommends taking fenugreek until you can smell it on your skin (or three capsules each of fenugreek and blessed thistle, taken three times a day). He notes that you'll usually see an increase in breast milk within the first 24 hours after taking these herbs. If you don't see a difference after a week, they may not be for you.
- Try to get more sleep. Call on friends and family to come over and watch baby for a couple of hours so you can have a nap, or go to bed early two to three nights a week.
- Reduce your stress. Having a baby can be stressful without all the usual demands in life. Stress can really impede breast milk production. Plan some relaxation time for yourself—ask someone to watch your baby while you take a long bath, get a massage, or curl up with a good book!

- Consult your doctor for medications that might help, or see the Newman Breastfeeding Clinic and Institute website for helpful breastfeeding information sheets (www.nbci.ca).

BREASTFEEDING AND SOLID FOOD

When your baby reaches six months of age, it's time to start him on solid food. Some mothers decide to put off giving their children solids and breastfeed only for the first year. I have yet to hear of any health concerns in any children who were exclusively breastfed for their first year.

Your baby has been exposed to many different tastes and flavours through your breast milk—when you eat spicy food, for instance, or garlic and onions. Most babies enjoy the flavour and spice, but it can also go the other way. You may recall a time when you ate a spicy curry or Thai meal and your baby was up all night! Exposure to moderate spices not only helps everyone sleep at night, but is a good start to the new experience of eating food.

When your baby first starts solids, her breast milk intake shouldn't change. As her appetite for solid food increases to two or three meals a day, she might nurse less, although you may not even notice at first. She'll nurse a few minutes less here and there, until she drops a feeding altogether. But go easy on the amount of food—you don't want to take away the great nutrition of breast milk by offering too much food too quickly. Remember that everything your baby needs is in breast milk—especially in comparison to a few tablespoons of purée.

Natalie Rogers notes that "as the baby breast feeds less when solid foods are introduced, the milk becomes more concentrated in some minerals and proteins." It's nature's way of making sure that baby is still getting what he needs. I find that remarkable.

PUMPING AND STORING BREAST MILK

Pumping in the early days is usually an easy task and will give you milk to store for feedings when you're not around. Milk can be pumped and frozen in ice cube trays or in safe, sterile plastic bags designed for breast milk, which usually have lines to indicate the amount and a space to write the date so you can use the oldest first and know how long it's been in the freezer. Natalie Rogers gave me the rundown of storage: Milk can be stored in amounts that the baby will use in one feeding; pumped milk should be refrigerated within six hours and consumed within two to five days (shake to remix). If milk is frozen in a fridge freezer, use within one month, if in a deep freezer, use with six months. Discard any thawed and warmed milk that's leftover from the feeding. Warming should *never* be done in a microwave, as it creates hot spots and kills a lot of the delicate nutrients, immune components, and proteins. Try placing a milk-filled bottle or container in a bowl of very warm tap water or thawing it under running water, and warm to skin temperature. Never thaw milk overnight on the counter, as this enables bacteria in the milk to multiply. Don't use a stove to warm the milk—overheating can destroy the vitamin C content and alter the proteins, including the IgA.

WEANING

Breastfeeding can continue as long as you want it to. I recommend breastfeeding for the first two years, and even longer if possible, or at least regularly for the first year. If you're heading back to work around the time your baby turns one, offer the breast first thing in the morning and before bed (but don't forget to start brushing those baby teeth). Keeping the morning and evening breastfeed provides a time of closeness that's especially precious now, with the new dynamic of mom being away from baby. And if your one-year-old is off to daycare, she'll benefit from the extra immune protection, which she'll typically need!

When you feel that it's time to stop breastfeeding, you need to provide an alternative until your baby is at least one year old. Some doctors recommend giving cow's milk if your baby stops breastfeeding between 10 and 12 months, but I disagree. With cow's milk being the most allergenic food, it's better to wait until at least one year before giving it to your baby. At 10 months, your baby might still be drinking a lot, and four to six 237 mL (8 oz) bottles of cow's milk is a lot to digest. So the better option is to start on formula if you're weaning off breast milk before age one. This decision should also take into account the amount of solid food your baby is eating. See Chapter 11 for suggestions of milks to move on to at age one.

Mothers who are heading back to work after maternity leave are often anxious about weaning their babies from the breast before the big day. I've spoken with moms of six-month-olds who are already worrying, even though they're not heading back until their babies turn one. The amount of breastfeeding at 6 months is very different from that at 11 months. Wait until closer to 10 months to assess the situation so you can see how much your baby is nursing. You may find that only one or two breastfeedings need to be replaced while you're away, so you might not need to wean until the final weeks before you go back to work.

Trying to get your baby to take a bottle of anything can often be challenging, especially if mom is the one doing the feeding. Your baby might be wondering why, when the breast is right there, she has to drink from a bottle. It's better to have dad start feeding with a bottle to get your baby used to it (so she won't smell your milk); a skilled child-care worker also should be able to get a bottle or sippy cup full of some kind of milk into your baby, perhaps not on the first day, but it will come. I would encourage good eating habits—if your baby is eating food with varied nutrients, you won't need to worry as much about the milk.

I've known babies who refused to drink anything other than breast milk. It didn't matter what the other stuff came in—bottle, sippy cup, glass, or straw—they just weren't having it. Not all babies like the taste of milk or formula after breast milk, so if they won't take it, don't force it. If you're concerned about the lack of nutrients or calcium with respect to dairy, be more aware of the nutrients in food and what should be on the plate to make up for the lack of milk (see "Building Strong Bones" in Chapter 3 for calcium-rich foods). And those babies I know who refused the moo-juice have grown up just fine.

To wean your baby off the breast, start to offer the alternative by replacing one feed at a time about a month before you want to completely stop to balance your milk supply and to gradually introduce formula to baby's digestion. Don't be disappointed if you don't get instant success. Talk to your baby about what is coming up: "Mommy is going back to work and instead of nursing, this is what you are going to have when you are at ——, or when —— is here with you." Although they can't talk, babies need to know what's going on and why. You might also try shortening the time of each nursing and offering substitutions of either food or water. Let your baby know he'll still have nurses when he wakes up and before he goes to bed.

If you won't be physically away from your baby but just want to stop breastfeeding, distraction is the name of the game. When your baby wants to nurse and needs the nourishment, offer the breast. If the nursing is just for comfort, try to distract her with another activity. And again, talk to your baby about what's going on by explaining that nurses (or whatever you call them) are slowing down now, so here's what the alternative is. When my second daughter was finishing up nursing at 26 months, I talked with her about how she was just going to have a "little nurse" before bed. She would look up at me with those big baby-blue eyes and say, "Just a little nurse, Mommy," and slowly it happened less and less often. Dad got more involved in putting her to bed, so breastfeeding wasn't an issue. And to stop the morning nurse, dad would go to her and take her downstairs for breakfast, avoiding me and the usual morning routine. At this age, she had started multi-tasking nursing—while latched on to my breast, she flipped her body around, put one leg in the air, and inflicted other torturous acts on my poor breasts. I and my nipples had had enough breastfeeding gymnastics!

One of the moms who attended my Mommy Chef cooking classes nursed her daughter for the first year. Her doctor was worried that the baby was not gaining enough weight, as she wasn't eating much solid food. So she suggested that mom stop breastfeeding almost immediately. The mom called me to talk about it, and I suggested that it wasn't the breast milk that was stopping her baby from eating, but rather the fact that she just wasn't a big eater. But mom wasn't convinced, so she took matters into her own hands. She went to the medicine cabinet, took out four Band-Aids, and covered her nipples with an X. The daughter co-slept with mom and dad, so she usually had an all-night buffet. When she saw the Band-Aids, mom talked to her about how the "nurses" were all gone. The daughter was not too happy about it, and apparently kept checking to see if mom's breasts were still bandaged up, but after the second day, she came to accept it. Mom was really engorged and had to pump, but that was that—her baby was weaned. Her daughter did put on a few extra pounds initially, and although she still isn't a big eater, she's really healthy!

5

MORE WHITE STUFF
Formula-Feeding

I fully endorse breastfeeding of babies and toddlers, and I wish that every child could be given the remarkable benefits of breast milk. Over the years I've met many mothers who wished they could breastfeed and tried everything to nurse their babies, but sometimes it just doesn't work out. A lactation consultant can offer incredible support (see the Resources for ways to get help). Even if you can't offer breast milk exclusively, don't despair—any amount of breast milk that you did give your baby has him off to a great start. If you nursed for the first few days in the hospital and he received colostrum, well done! If you breastfed for six weeks, three months, or nine months, even better.

Some moms choose not to breastfeed or to nurse only some of the time or for a shorter period. Others don't have a choice—they may not be able to offer any breast milk at all due to complications during labour and delivery,

> ### From the Mouths of Moms
> I was never truly comfortable with breastfeeding. I always had trouble getting into the right position or breastfeeding in public, and my son would take an hour and a half to eat and would still be hungry. Ultimately, I persevered for six months (also supplementing with formula) because I knew the benefits that it would give him. Breastfeeding to this day stresses me out, but I would definitely do it over again—I'd just ask for more help next time.
> —KATIE, MOM OF ONE

because they adopted or had a surrogate carry their child, and for many other reasons. Many babies who've grown up on formula milk are fit and healthy. And being informed when it comes to purchasing an infant formula can give you greater confidence in your choice and help to alleviate the guilt that can overwhelm some moms.

CHOOSING THE RIGHT FORMULA

You'll need to know the ins and outs of formula before choosing which one is right for your little one—remember, every baby is different. Your doctor may recommend brands when you're thinking about starting formula. However, formula company salespeople inform doctors about their products, and your doctor might not have asked for the same information that you would have. I'd be overjoyed if some of these questions were answered—such as "Does your product contain genetically modified ingredients?" or "What research have you done into the possible negative effects of MSG (monosodium glutamate), which is in your hydrolyzed formula?" or even "How confident are you about the DHA source in this formula? I've heard that it can cause diarrhea in some babies"—but that's not very realistic.[47] In fact, while I was researching this section, it proved difficult, if not impossible, to get responses to my own questions from the formula companies.

There can be many influences on your decision about which formula to purchase, and although health care professionals are the right place to start, it's best to keep searching until you're confident that you've made an informed choice.

Survey Says ... Formula-Buying Influences

In an online survey, I asked moms why they chose a particular formula. Of the 216 moms who responded, 39 percent used a formula recommended by their doctor; 25 percent chose the one used in the hospital; 19 percent used one recommended by a professional (other than a doctor); 28 percent said that a friend told them about it; 15 percent bought organic; 40 percent chose a formula with DHA; 15 percent used one with extra iron; 2 percent bought because it was soy; and 1 percent said they liked the packaging.[48]

FORMULA MARKETING

Infant formula is big business. A lot of money goes into its marketing, and the competition is stiff. There are about 10 main formula companies in Canada and the United States, all wanting your dollars. At The Baby Time Show, where I exhibit twice a year in Toronto, the booths and displays of the formula makers are enormous and are always packed with attendees receiving their leaflets and free samples. These companies can be very persuasive in claiming that their product is the most like breast milk—this may be true, but it all depends on which aspects they're comparing. The most recent additions to formula are DHA, AA, and some beneficial bacteria, all of which, manufacturers note, makes it "closest to breast milk." But what about the rest of what it may be missing? Keep in mind that the companies are in it for the sales, not necessarily for your best interests.

With so many brands, types, and categories of formula on the market, browsing the formula aisle in the supermarket, drugstore, or even health food store can be overwhelming. You might be saying to yourself, "High in iron ... that sounds good—iron is important, right? And that one has DHA and AA—not sure what they are, but the formula companies know what they're doing so it must be OK ... I think."

Deciding on a formula for your baby should involve careful consideration. There are good reasons for choosing one formula over another, and it's not about the catchy labelling. Your baby may need a certain protein ratio or need the proteins broken down a bit (known as hydrolyzed), you might prefer an organic formula (I know I would!), or maybe you're unsure what any of it means or what might be right for your baby. So let's start at the beginning and look at some of the most common ingredients in formula.

It's Your Choice

Whatever the reason you're reading this chapter, you may not be breast-feeding by choice. Whether you have low milk production or need to increase your baby's weight (although in some cases, formula-feeding may not be what's best for your baby), if you feel your doctor isn't supportive enough of your wish to breastfeed, find a lactation consultant who can help (see the Resources).

Formula Ingredients: The Good and the Not So Good

Protein

The protein source in dairy formulas is whey and/or casein. The ratio of whey to casein seems to differ among the formulas suitable for different age groups. Newborn formula has a ratio of whey to casein similar to breast milk, and those for six-month-olds and older babies offer different proportions. If your baby is displaying any symptoms of allergic reaction—eczema, asthma, blood in the stool, vomiting or hives—it's mostly caused by the beta lactoglobulin protein in whey (only protein is associated with type 1 allergy—see Chapter 7). Some babies and children, especially autistic children, have difficulty digesting casein. See the table comparing various formulas' ingredients on page 92.

Soy formula relies on the soybean as its protein source. Soy formula is advised in the case of galactosemia (a rare genetic metabolic disorder) or an allergy to cow's milk (although hydrolyzed formula may be a better option). See below for more on soy formula.

Carbohydrates

Lactose, maltodextrin, corn syrup, sucrose, and brown rice syrup are carbohydrates added to formula for energy as well as sweetness. Because lactose is also found in breast milk, most babies will tolerate it well and it's the best choice of carbohydrate. Corn syrup, brown rice syrup, and sucrose are used in place of lactose. Corn syrup and sucrose are worrisome, as nonorganic corn syrup may contain genetically modified corn, and sucrose is a simple sugar and so can lead to a sweet tooth.

In an interview I conducted with Jay Highman, the founder of Nature's One, the manufacturer of Baby's Only Organic formula, he explained that lactose is naturally occurring in all milk powder used for formula unless it's taken out. "So when lactose is listed in the ingredient declaration panel," Highman explains, "this means an additional amount of lactose has been added to complete the carbohydrate requirements of a baby. The added amount of lactose can overwhelm a baby's available supply of lactase, an enzyme found in the small intestine needed to break down milk lactose. If there is not enough lactase, then undigested lactose moves into the intestinal tract and produces bloating, cramps, diarrhea and ultimately a very unhappy baby. Baby's Only Organic daily formula does not list lactose as an ingredient because it's naturally occurring. We complete the carbohydrate requirement by adding a complex carbohydrate, organic brown rice syrup. We believe that is the perfect balance." Formula manufacturers are required to list anything that's been added to formula. Nature's One formulas include brown rice syrup, an easily digested source of carbohydrates that's more complex than sucrose, for instance, in its carbohydrate structure; it enters the bloodstream slowly, as lactose does, but without stressing the lactase enzyme. This is called a low glycemic food, and it's preferable for everyone's blood sugar stability.

Fats

Soybean, high oleic (acid), sunflower, safflower, palm olein, and coconut oil are all found on the ingredient lists of formulas and make up the fatty acids your baby needs. Formula companies use a mixture of a variety of these oils to create a fatty acid profile closest to that of breast milk. Some research indicates that palm olein oil is not preferred because it's associated with constipation.[49] Another study concluded that "healthy term infants fed a formula containing PO (palm olein) as the predominant oil in the fat blend had significantly lower BMC (bone mineral content) and BMD (bone mineral density) than those fed a formula without PO. The inclusion of PO in infant formula at levels needed to provide a fatty acid profile similar to that of human milk leads to lower bone mineralization."[50]

Avoiding palm olein oil might narrow down your choices considerably—I came across only two formulas that didn't have it, one of which isn't widely available in Canada. Other formulas listed "palm oil or palm olein," making it difficult to know for sure which oil is included. It irks me when manufacturers use "or." I understand that the supply of certain ingredient may be limited so they're hedging their bets on what they can get, but especially in the case of formula, I want to know exactly what's in the product. If you do use formula with palm olein oil, counteract constipation with extra probiotics and flax seed oil until you find an alternative (see Chapter 6 for more on constipation).

Iron

Formula must contain minerals within a set range, so you'll notice that the nutritional content of all formulas is roughly the same. One of the most important minerals during infancy is iron, as it's involved in brain development and cognitive function. All formula is fortified with a level of between 0.7 and 1.2 mg iron per 100 mL. When deciding whether your baby needs a higher level of iron or not, you'll need to take your baby's history into consideration. For instance, was your baby premature? If so, look for a formula that's a bit higher in iron because premies are more likely to have lower iron stores (they didn't have the time in utero to take what they needed from you). Note that there are formulas for premature babies with an easier-to-absorb protein structure. If your baby was born at term and had a low birth weight (under 2.5 kg, or 5 lb, 5 oz), you may also want to consider a formula with a bit more iron. For all other babies, a higher than average iron-fortified formula isn't necessary.

The big concern with iron is its absorbability. Breast milk contains two proteins, lactoferrin and transferrin, which grab on to the iron, delivering it to your baby's bloodstream and keeping any bad bacteria in the intestines from making a meal of it (bad bacteria thrive on iron). Formula doesn't contain these key proteins. So you'll need to assess whether your baby is likely to have high levels of bad bacteria in her intestines (we all have a certain amount). Look back at your pregnancy, labour and delivery, and postpartum period if you were breastfeeding. If you took antibiotics during any of these times, it's possible that your baby will have lower levels of good bacteria to keep the bad guys in check. If your baby was given antibiotics or was born by Caesarean section, the same applies. When more bad bacteria are hanging around, there's less chance for your baby to absorb iron from the formula. So offer a human strain of probiotics or beneficial bacteria containing *Bifidobacterium infantis* and *Lactobacillus acidophilus* at a level of three billion bacteria twice daily after a feeding. This should help to keep the bad bacteria at bay and therefore allow iron to be better absorbed.

Essential Fatty Acids

Essential fatty acids—DHA and AA (or ARA)—are a newer addition to formula. DHA and AA are essential for the development of the brain, eye, and nervous systems. Formula companies are marketing this addition as making their products that much closer to breast milk, leading parents to believe that formula is as good as breast milk, which is not, in fact, the case. These added fats have also created controversy. In a 2008 report, the Cornucopia Institute, an organization in support of sustainable and organic agriculture, examined the use of these oils in formula.[51] The institute's concern is that DHA and AA are extracted from algae and fungal sources and processed using a toxic chemical. The report also commented on formula companies' financial gain from marketing formula with these oils in it. The main worry, though, was that these oils can cause diarrhea in babies, leading to health complications. It's a tough decision whether to buy formula fortified with these essential fatty acids. I have suggested to some parents that they purchase formula without the DHA and AA and add the DHA themselves. Babies can use the other fats in formula to make AA in their bodies, but they can't do the same for DHA in the level they need for optimal brain and eye development. And, of course, the exact composition of DHA and AA

Survey Says ... Purchasing Influences

In my online survey of 216 moms, 40 percent said they chose a formula because it was fortified with DHA and AA, and 39 percent said their purchase was influenced by their doctor's recommendation.

in breast milk may not resemble that added to formula. That said, some research conducted on small groups of children has shown an increase in IQ and visual acuity in babies fed formula fortified with DHA and AA.[52] *An important note:* Do not give babies under six months any supplement containing the omega-3 fatty acid EPA (eicosapentaenoic acid), as it competes with AA for absorption.

Nucleotides

Nucleotides are molecules that help make up the structure of DNA and RNA (ribonucleic acid) and are naturally found in breast milk. Some formula companies (mostly in the United States) have been adding nucleotides to their formula for several years. At a time of such rapid growth and cell turnover in your baby's digestive, immune, and metabolic cells, nucleotides are important factors.

Beneficial Bacteria

One formula company (at the time of writing) has added in "Natural Cultures," or probiotics. Good bacteria are so important for your baby's digestive and immune systems, and although this formula has only one strain, *Bifidobacterium lactis,* it's a good start. My concern is that most probiotics need to be refrigerated and will die off with any heat, so how much will be left after warming formula (especially if warmed in a microwave) and even after opening the tin?

TYPES OF FORMULA

Soy Formula

Soy formula may be the only choice for some babies, such as those with the rare genetic disorder galactosemia or cow's milk allergy (although some babies who are allergic to dairy are also allergic to soy). "The American Academy of Pediatrics states that soy protein-based formula is a *reasonable* alternative for term infants who cannot tolerate cow milk-based formulas or lactose found in cow's milk formulas."[53]

When buying soy formula, go with an organic one. Almost all conventional soy is genetically modified (GM) and may lead to negative health issues. GM soy (canola, cotton, and corn) is a product that I advise all parents to avoid, whether in the form of tofu, tempeh, soy sauce, edamame (soybeans in their shells), milk, or formula. The potential health risks include higher chances of developing allergies because the DNA structure of the food has been altered and becomes similar to other allergens or the GM food has been adulterated with a part of a nut, such as Brazil nut in the case of some soy products.[54] Babies and toddlers have such fast growth rates in their first years that they have much greater susceptibility to health issues from eating GM foods.[55] Check out www.geneticroulette.com for research as well as up-to-date lists about which foods contain GM ingredients. Conventional or nonorganic dairy formula also has the potential to contain GM products from corn and from the cows being fed GM feed, affecting their milk. It takes a bit of research to find out which foods may contain GM products, but once you look into the issue, you'll understand why the extra effort is worth it.

Another reason to be cautious of consuming any soy product, whether organic or conventional, is that soy contains a compound called phytate. Phytate binds with minerals such as iron, zinc, and calcium and interferes with their absorption by the body. Although soy formula is fortified with these minerals, as well as phosphorus, it's not recommended for premature babies as it has been associated with a higher risk of low bone density (osteopenia).[56] But for all other babies, soy formula may be the only option.

Goat's Milk Formula

Nanny Care Goat Milk Formula is worth mentioning here. I recommended this formula while practising in England, and when I moved back to Canada I was most disappointed to find that it isn't available here. It's produced in New Zealand by the Dairy Goat Co-operative and is available throughout the United Kingdom. This is the only formula I've found that really offers superior absorbability and ease of digestion, and clears up all sorts of reactions, including eczema, spitting up, behaviour issues, and colic. The company notes on its website some

From the Mouths of Moms (or an Aunt, in This Case)

Jonathan was breastfed until his mom got the flu when he was seven months old. Mom was so sick that he went to stay with his grandparents and was given formula. He tried different formulas, and eventually the parents decided to give him soy, since they were following a vegan diet. Mom couldn't return to breastfeeding, as she had stopped producing milk while Jonathan was away. Jonathan's sleep pattern changed after starting the formula, but mom and dad put it down to the different situation of changing from breast milk to a bottle. He drank soy formula until he was 13 months old and then switched to soy milk and sometimes almond milk. When he was 15 months, mom and dad went on holiday and left Jonathan with the grandparents again. His diet was altered and he didn't have any soy at all—no milk, tofu, veggie burgers, or hot dogs—for almost two weeks. The first time he drank soy milk again was one night before bed, and the family noticed that he was tossing and turning more than usual. About two hours after he had fallen asleep, Jonathan began crying. I ran to his bedside and saw him violently thrashing his legs, then curling up into a ball and stretching out, as if he couldn't find a comfortable position. I noticed that Jonathan was still asleep but was crying as if he had fallen and hurt himself. I lifted Jonathan and tried walking with him to soothe him. He couldn't stay still. Then I noticed that the gas that Jonathan passed smelled unusual—toxic is the best way to describe it. The parents couldn't quite believe that this could be a reaction to soy, so a few days later they tried it again, and the same thing happened. He now avoids all soy products and will do so for a long time.

—BETTY, AUNT OF JONATHAN

benefits of this formula: It offers a protein source that's easier to digest (smaller curds), supports digestive health by reducing "leaky gut," contains absorbable fatty acids, is made from the milk of goats that are naturally raised without growth stimulants and hormones, has essential nutrients needed for growth, and if you are so inclined, can even be used in cooking![57]

I often recommend goat's milk as a substitute for dairy for toddlers over one year of age; it seems to be less reactive than cow's milk. But some still react, so it's not for everyone. If you're at your wits' end looking for a formula that's less reactive or a better product, try to think of someone in the United Kingdom who can order Nanny Care and ship it to you, or find an online retailer—I'm confident that it will help your baby. Even if you use it for a short time while you sort out another less expensive alternative (shipping cost is usually high) or use it in rotation with another formula, it at least gives you an option.

Lactose-Free Formula

When I first heard of lactose-free formula, I wondered what on earth the formula companies were up to now. Breast milk contains lactose, so it's almost impossible for babies to be lactose intolerant. But after hearing from parents how much better their babies did on lactose-free formula, I did some further research.

Lactose is the sugar, or carbohydrate, most commonly found in all milk, from both humans and animals. Not only is it an important carbohydrate source, but it enhances calcium absorption and helps the colonization of good bacteria in baby's intestines.

All babies are born with the enzyme *lactase* to digest the *lactose*. In very rare instances, a congenital defect prevents lactase production. Premature babies may be born with low levels of lactase production and might benefit from a lactose-free formula as their lactase levels reach 70 percent by 34th to 35th week.[58] Otherwise, in most children, lactase enzyme production slows around age two or three, and symptoms of gas and bloating, loose stools, abdominal cramps with discomfort, and nausea may show up at about five to six years. Symptoms often depend on the amount and type of dairy consumed. Our bodies were made to take in milk (usually breast milk) for the first two or so years of life and then to get our nutrients from food. Cow's milk isn't really meant for humans, but somehow we have adapted to be able to drink or eat dairy products. Milk is usually the least tolerated dairy product, since its lactose level is higher than in other dairy products. And in certain situations, lactase production may be unable to keep up with the amount of lactose ingested, such as when a baby quickly drinks large amounts of formula every day. Any formula with lactose on the ingredient list has more than a naturally occurring level and may overwhelm the lactase enzyme.

Secondary lactose intolerance can be caused by digestive disorders such as celiac disease, gastroenteritis, or diarrhea (even from teething). There may be damage to the enzyme-producing sites in the intestines, or the enzyme may be *whooshed* out in cases of diarrhea as the body tries to get rid of bacteria, a virus, or a parasite. In any case of diarrhea, whatever the cause, it's advisable to remove

dairy from the diet immediately. If
your baby is on formula, switch to a
lactose-free formula to avoid lactose
intolerance and the symptoms
described below. Once the diarrhea
episode has passed, wait three days
before returning to your baby's usual
formula. If gassy symptoms start, be
sure that you're giving probiotics, and
slowly ease back on to the usual formula, rather than making a straight switch.

> ### Cow's Milk Is *for Their Babies*
> Cow's milk is produced for calves,
> large animals that need a particular
> set of nutrients proportionate to
> their bodies. Calves weigh between
> 80 and 100 pounds at birth and
> generally wean themselves by nine
> months.

Lactose-free formulas replace the lactose with corn syrup, sucrose, or brown
rice syrup. As I mentioned above, the use of corn syrup is a concern because it
can be made of GM corn, it's very sweet, and it has been associated with allergies.
Sucrose also isn't the best choice because it's as sweet as purple grape juice and
can lead to overfeeding.[59] Search out an organic formula that uses an alternative
sweetener or carbohydrate.

Common symptoms of lactose intolerance are diarrhea, gassiness, and colic-
like pain and fussiness. If you see these symptoms in your baby, a lactose-free formula might be the right one for her.

Hydrolyzed Formula

Hydrolyzed formula predigests or breaks down the proteins to make them more
digestible, and so this is often the product of choice for babies showing symptoms of milk allergy.

One drawback with hydrolyzed formula is that the process of predigesting the
protein to amino acids results in a bitter taste, so ingredients are added to
improve it. Also during this process, the lactose is taken out and replaced with a
carbohydrate source and a sweetener, usually corn syrup or sucrose. As well, the
benefits of lactose in helping with the absorption of calcium and the replication
or reproduction of good bacteria in the intestines are lost.

Hydrolyzed formulas are sometimes recommended to prevent milk allergy,
as it's the proteins in milk that usually cause an allergy. I'd suggest looking into
a hydrolyzed formula if your baby has a higher potential for allergies because he
has a sibling with an anaphylactic food allergy; he wasn't breastfed at all; he was

born by Caesarean section; you took antibiotics during pregnancy, during labour and delivery, or while breastfeeding; your baby has had antibiotics; or there's a family history of allergy in either parents or a sibling. Use hydrolyzed formula while you support the digestive system with probiotics for at least one month, then switch to a nonhydrolized one.

Hydrolyzed formula isn't offered as an organic product, and it's usually more expensive than nonhydrolyzed formula. So far, only three brands are available in Canada. But I've seen this formula help many babies who couldn't tolerate the other types—babies who were once gassy and uncomfortable, waking through the night, sometimes sleep better, and eczema can improve (although infant probiotics often give better results).

The outcomes of babies who are given hydrolyzed formula for a prolonged period of time haven't been studied in depth, but some parents may have no choice but to use it.

Premixed or Powder

Premixed formulas may be a better option for premature babies because of the risks of not mixing powder formula properly or contaminating it with bacteria on mixing. However, avoid premixed formula until the companies switch to can linings that are free from bisphenol A (BPA), a toxin commonly used in plastic and by-products that's associated with increased risk of breast and prostate cancer and is neurotoxic to infants during development. Sterilizing your bottles; letting them air-dry; using filtered, boiled, and cooled water to make up the powder formula; and double-checking your measurements should eliminate any problems with powder formula. The cans of powder formula also contain BPA, but powder appears to have less leaching potential. Premixed formula might be a better choice if you're going away on holiday and can't guarantee the cleanliness of the water. Finally, although premixed formula can be convenient, it's usually more expensive.

THE BOTTOM LINE: DO YOUR RESEARCH

Step 1:   Before choosing your formula, check for recent recalls or contamination information on the websites for the Canadian Food Inspection Agency (www.inspection.gc.ca) and the U.S. Food and Drug Administration (www.fda.gov). The last thing you want is to find out that your formula has been recalled or found to contain something that it shouldn't.

Step 2: Next, check the Environmental Working Group website (www.ewg.org) for the latest on BPA in the lining of formula tins or cans. EWG says that currently, premixed formula contains more BPA than powdered formula. Although recently attention has been given to banning BPA in baby bottles, the focus doesn't seem to have been on formula cans—yet. This may also help you decide which product to buy.

Step 3: Consider whether to go organic or not. I'd highly recommend buying an organic formula. There are three on the Canadian market, and more in the United States. I have had clients who had Baby's Only Organic formula delivered from the United States to their homes. At the time of writing, Baby's Only Organic was sold in one store in Toronto and could also be purchased online (see reference section). I much prefer its ingredient list to that of other organic formulas, and I like how the company promotes breastfeeding until one year; the labels say the formula is for toddlers, although it's suitable from birth. Although some organic formulas' ingredient lists aren't perfect, buying organic lessens the possibility of exposure to the hormones, antibiotics, and GM feed given to cows and reduces the overall toxic load from herbicides and pesticides.

Step 4: If your baby seems to be having a problem with formula and shows signs of spitting up, diarrhea or constipation, eczema, or rashes; doesn't sleep well; seems restless and unsettled (different from poor sleep habits); or is failing to develop or gain weight as expected, first speak with your doctor about these issues, and then see the table comparing formulas at the end of the chapter or check your ingredient list. Don't discount the possibility that a health issue may be linked to formula. Look at the ingredients list, not the nutrition information, and see what the sweetener or carbohydrate source is—lactose, corn, or something else (brown rice syrup is less likely to cause a problem). Then look at the protein source— whey or casein or a mix of both. Breast milk is a mix of both proteins in a ratio of about 70 percent whey to 30 percent casein, so both are important. If your baby is suffering from constipation, look for palm olein oil on the label. If it's there, find another brand (Similac and Nature's One have no palm olein oil). Steer away from extra iron (remember, all formulas are fortified with iron) if your baby was born at term or later and hasn't had any bleeding or blood tests, especially if you're not giving probiotics. If you don't go with a formula with added DHA and AA, supplement with DHA only (no EPA) until six months (Genestra's Super Neurogen DHA is 200 mg DHA only from an algae source, lessening the potential for allergic reaction). After six months, a DHA and EPA mix can be given, but remember that it comes from fish, so if your baby has the potential for allergies, introduce it slowly. Try to find a capsule form and bite a hole in it, then squeeze the contents into your baby's mouth once a day after a bottle.

Step 5: No matter which formula you choose, *always* give probiotics. This should help with iron absorption as well as reduce the risk of allergies and support the maturation of the digestive system. Probiotics are suitable for any baby.

Step 6: If your baby has no particular health issues, don't get too fancy. A standard formula (again, preferably organic) is just fine. Formula has been around for years, and dairy formula is the oldest and most trusted (although I prefer Nanny Care Goat Milk Formula). Unless absolutely necessary, avoid soy formula, but if you have to use it, buy organic (Nature's One/Baby's Only). Formula companies are continually improving their products and seem committed to providing the best product they can. In years to come it wouldn't surprise me to see probiotics in all infant formulas, but, as usual, there will probably be some controversy over the source, type, and strain.

Step 7: Be a savvy shopper. Read your ingredients and shop around. Although there's a certain stigma to buying the chain stores' generic brands or products, comparing their ingredient labels with those of the top brands may save you a lot of money. In my research of different formulas, organic and conventional, I saw a lot of similarities in ingredients that led me to dig deeper. I found out that one company manufactures formula products for many retail companies (especially the organic ones), which then put their own private labels. There can be up to fifteen dollars' difference in price for the same product. Another good reason to read your label and compare products: if they look the same, they are the same.

I believe that the greater incidence of allergy is partly to do with babies being fed formula with the new ingredients described in this chapter, some from genetically modified sources, and this worries me a lot. We won't know for years what the negative effects of these new formulas might be, until there's an increase in a certain disease or a new illness that affects our children's generation. All you can do is to make an informed choice by doing your research and asking the important questions, and then lift the weight of guilt off your shoulders, knowing that you've done the best that you can. That's great parenting!

Tips for Mixing Powder Formula

- To reduce the risk of bacteria contamination, sterilize your bottles and always wash your hands before preparing the formula.
- Let the bottles air-dry before filling them.
- Use filtered water that is boiled and cooled. Reverse osmosis filtered water can be used straight from the tap or bottle (I'd suggest boiling it for premies or newborns, though).
- Check the expiry date on the can.
- Carefully follow the instructions for quantity of water to powder, and once mixed, refrigerate and use within 24 hours.
- If you're going out, bring a bottle with pre-measured dry powder and mix it with water from a thermos (to keep it warm), rather than taking an already mixed bottle. That way, you don't need to keep the formula cool while you're out and about.
- Discard immediately anything your baby doesn't drink from a prepared bottle.

CANADIAN FORMULA COMPARISON CHART WITH SWEETENER, IRON, AND FATS

	Protein Source	Sweetener Type	Iron Content	Fat Type	DHA/ARA Nucleotide, and Probiotic Fortification	Pricing and Size
NON-FORTIFIED FORMULAS						
Similac Regular	Casein and whey	Lactose	Fe=0.47 mg/ 100 mL	High oleic sunflower oil, coconut oil, soy oil	Nucleotides	$25.29 900 g
Enfamil Lower Iron	Casein and whey	Corn syrup and lactose	Fe=0.74 mg/ 100 mL	Palm olein, soy oil, high oleic sunflower oil	None	$24.99 730 g
Nanny Care Goat Milk Formula	Casein and whey	Lactose	Fe=0.85 mg/ 100 mL	Canola and sunflower oil	None	Available only in UK and New Zealand
FORTIFIED FORMULAS						
Similac Advance with DHA and ARA	Casein and whey	Lactose	Fe=1.2 mg/ 100 mL	High oleic sunflower oil, coconut oil, soy oil	DHA=5 mg/ 100 mL ARA=13 mg/ 100 mL Nucleotides	$29.99 900 g
Similac Iron Fortified	Casein and whey	Lactose	Fe=1.2 mg/ 100 mL	High oleic sunflower oil, coconut oil, soy oil	Nucleotides	$23.99 900 g
Similac Step 2 Go & Grow	Casein and whey	Lactose	Fe=1.2 mg/ 100 mL	High oleic sunflower oil, coconut oil, soy oil	Nucleotides	$25.99 900 g
Similac Step 2 Go & Grow with Omega-3 & 6	Casein and whey	Lactose	Fe=1.2 mg/ 100 mL	High oleic sunflower oil, coconut oil, soy oil	DHA=5 mg/ 100 mL ARA=14 mg/ 100 mL Nucleotides	$31.89 728 g

continued

	Protein Source	Sweetener Type	Iron Content	Fat Type	DHA/ARA Nucleotide, and Probiotic Fortification	Pricing and Size
Nestlé Good Start Stage 1 with Omega-3 & 6 and Natural Cultures	Whey	Lactose	Fe=1 mg/ 100 mL	Palm olein, soybean oil, coconut oil	DHA=10 mg/ 100 mL ARA=20 mg/ 100 mL Nucleotides and *Bifidobacterium lactis*	$33.99 640 g
Nestlé Good Start Stage 1	Whey	Lactose	Fe=1 mg/ 100 mL	Palm olein, soybean oil, coconut oil	None	$25.29 900 g
Heinz Nurture Stage 1 with Omega-3 & 6	Casein and whey	Lactose	Fe=1.2 mg/ 100 mL	Palm oil or palm olein, soy oil, high oleic sunflower or safflower oil, coconut oil	DHA=5.7 mg/ 100 mL ARA=9.8 mg/ 100 mL	$25.99 730 g
Heinz Nurture Stage 2 with Omega-3 & 6	Casein and whey	Lactose	Fe=1.2 mg/ 100 mL	Palm oil or palm olein, soy oil, high oleic sunflower or safflower oil, coconut oil nucleotides	DHA=11.6 mg/ 100 mL ARA=23.2 mg/ 100 mL	$24.99 730 g
PC Infant Formula (Dairy) (Loblaws)	Casein and whey	Lactose	Fe=1.2 mg/ 100 mL	High oleic sunflower or safflower oil, coconut oil, soy oil, palm olein	None	$15.39 900 g
Parent's Choice Milk Infant Formula with DHA and ARA (Walmart)	Casein and whey	Lactose	Fe=1.2 mg/ 100 mL	High oleic sunflower or safflower oil, coconut oil, soy oil, palm olein	DHA=5.7 mg/ 100 mL ARA=9.8 mg/ 100 mL	$21.97 1020 g

continued

CANADIAN FORMULA COMPARISON CHART WITH SWEETENER, IRON, AND FATS (continued)

	Protein Source	Sweetener Type	Iron Content	Fat Type	DHA/ARA Nucleotide, and Probiotic Fortification	Pricing and Size
Enfamil Lipil Iron Fortified	Casein and whey	Corn syrup and lactose	Fe=1.2 mg/ 100 mL	Palm olein, soy oil, high oleic sunflower oil	None	$24.99 1000 g
Enfamil A+ with DHA and ARA	Casein and whey	Corn syrup and lactose	Fe=1.2 mg/ 100 mL	Palm olein, soy oil, high oleic sunflower oil	DHA=11.5 mg/ 100 mL ARA=23 mg/ 100 mL	$29.99 730 g
Kirkland Signature with Omega-3 & 6 (Costco)	Casein and whey	Lactose	Fe=1.2 mg/ 100 mL	High oleic sunflower oil, coconut oil, soy oil	DHA and ARA Nucleotides	$17.89 900 g
SOY FORMULA						
Isomil Soy Formula Plus Iron	Soy	Corn syrup and sucrose	Fe=1.2 mg/ 100 mL	High oleic sunflower or safflower oil, coconut oil, soy oil	None	$31.99 800 g
Isomil Step 2	Soy	Corn syrup and sucrose	Fe=1.2 mg/ 100 mL	High oleic sunflower or safflower oil, coconut oil, soy oil	None	$26.39 800 g
Isomil Advance with Omega-3 & 6	Soy	Corn syrup and sucrose	Fe=1.2 mg/ 100 mL	High oleic sunflower or safflower oil, coconut oil, soy oil	DHA=5 mg/ 100 mL ARA=14 mg/ 100 mL	$31.99 800 g
Parent's Choice Soy Formula (Walmart)	Soy	Corn syrup	Fe=1.2 mg/ 100 mL	High oleic sunflower or safflower oil, coconut oil, soy oil, palm olein	None	$21.17 730 g

continued

	Protein Source	Sweetener Type	Iron Content	Fat Type	DHA/ARA Nucleotide, and Probiotic Fortification	Pricing and Size
Nestlé Alsoy with Omega-3 & 6	Soy	Sucrose	Fe=1.2 mg/ 100 mL	Palm olein, soybean oil, coconut oil	DHA=10 mg/ 100 mL ARA=20 mg/ 100 mL	$29.99 730 g
Enfamil Soy A+ with Omega-3 & 6	Soy	Corn syrup	Fe=1.2 mg/ 100 mL	Palm olein, soy oil, high oleic sunflower oil	DHA=11.5 mg/ 100 mL ARA=23 mg/ 100 mL	$29.99 730 g
PC Infant Formula (Soy) with Omega-3 & 6 (Loblaws)	Soy	Corn syrup	Fe=1.2 mg/ 100 mL	Palm olein, soy oil, high oleic sunflower oil, coconut oil	DHA=11.5 mg/ 100 mL ARA=23 mg/ 100 mL	$20.99 730 g
ORGANIC DAIRY FORMULAS						
Navita Organic with Omega-3 & 6 and Iron (Shoppers Drug Mart)	Casein and whey	Lactose	Fe=1.2 mg/ 100 mL	Organic palm oil or palm olein, organic soy oil, organic high oleic sunflower or safflower oil, organic coconut oil	DHA=10 mg/ 100 mL ARA=20 mg/ 100 mL	$26.99 730 g
PC Organics Infant Formula with Omega-3 & 6 (Loblaws)	Casein and whey	Lactose	Fe=1.2 mg/ 100 mL	Organic palm oil or palm olein, organic soy oil, organic high oleic sunflower or safflower oil, organic coconut oil	DHA=10 mg/ 100 mL ARA=20 mg/ 100 mL	$25.99 730 g

continued

CANADIAN FORMULA COMPARISON CHART WITH SWEETENER, IRON, AND FATS (continued)

	Protein Source	Sweetener Type	Iron Content	Fat Type	DHA/ARA Nucleotide, and Probiotic Fortification	Pricing and Size
Nature's One Baby's Only Organic	Casein and whey	Rice syrup	Fe=1.2 mg/ 100 mL	Organic high oleic sunflower oil, organic soybean oil, organic coconut oil	None	$15.00 360 g
Parent's Choice Organic Infant Formula	Casein and whey	Lactose	Fe=1.2 mg/ 100 mL	High oleic sunflower or safflower oil, coconut oil, soy oil, palm olein	DHA=10 mg/ 100 mL ARA=20 mg/ 100 mL	$21.97 730 g
My Organic Baby Dairy Formula	Casein and whey	Lactose	Fe=1.2 mg/ 100 mL	Organic palm oil or palm olein, organic soy oil, organic high oleic sunflower or safflower oil, organic coconut oil	DHA=10 mg/ 100 mL ARA=20 mg/ 100 mL	$33.99 730 g
ORGANIC SOY FORMULA						
PC Organics Soy Formula with Omega-3 & 6 (Loblaws)	Soy	Corn syrup	Fe=1.2 mg/ 100 mL	Organic palm oil or palm olein, organic soy oil, organic high oleic sunflower or safflower oil, organic coconut oil	DHA=11 mg/ 100 mL ARA=20 mg/ 100 mL	$25.99 730 g
My Organic Baby Soy with Omega-3 & 6	Soy	Corn syrup	Fe=1.2 mg/ 100 mL	Organic palm oil or palm olein, organic soy oil, organic high oleic sunflower or safflower oil, organic coconut oil	DHA=11 mg/ 100 mL ARA=20 mg/ 100 mL	$39.99 730 g

continued

	Protein Source	Sweetener Type	Iron Content	Fat Type	DHA/ARA Nucleotide, and Probiotic Fortification	Pricing and Size
Nature's One Baby's Only Organic Soy Formula	Soy	Rice syrup	Fe=1.2 mg/100 mL	Organic high oleic sunflower oil, organic soybean oil, organic coconut oil	None	$15.00 360 g
LACTOSE-FREE FORMULAS						
Similac Sensitive Lactose Free	Casein and whey	Sucrose	Fe=1.2 mg/100 mL	High oleic sunflower or safflower oil, coconut oil, soy oil	None	$31.89 728 g
Parent's Choice Gentle Infant Formula	Casein and whey	Corn syrup	Fe=1.2 mg/100 mL	High oleic sunflower or safflower oil, coconut oil, soy oil, palm olein	None	$19.77 730 g
Enfamil Lactose Free A+ with Omega-3 & 6	Casein and whey	Corn syrup	Fe=1.2 mg/100 mL	High oleic sunflower or safflower oil, coconut oil, soy oil, palm olein	DHA=11.5 mg/100 mL ARA=23 mg/100 mL	$31.89 730 g
ORGANIC LACTOSE-FREE FORMULAS						
Nature's One Baby's Only Lactose Free Formula	Casein and whey	Rice syrup	Fe=1.2 mg/100 mL	Organic high oleic sunflower oil, organic soybean oil, organic coconut oil	None	$19.50 360 g

continued

CANADIAN FORMULA COMPARISON CHART WITH SWEETENER, IRON, AND FATS (continued)

	Protein Source	Sweetener Type	Iron Content	Fat Type	DHA/ARA Nucleotide, and Probiotic Fortification	Pricing and Size
SPECIALTY FORMULAS						
Alimentum	Hydrolyzed casein	Sucrose	Fe=1.2 mg/ 100 mL	Safflower oil, MCT oil (fractionated coconut oil or palm kernel oil), soy oil	None	$7.49 Premixed only: 4 x 237 mL
Nutramigen A+	Hydrolyzed casein	Corn syrup	Fe=1.2 mg/ 100 mL	Palm olein, soy oil, coconut oil, high oleic sunflower oil	DHA=11.5 mg/ 100 mL ARA=23 mg/ 100 mL	$21.99 454 g
Enfamil Gentlease A+	Partially hydrolyzed casein and whey	Corn syrup	Fe=1.2 mg/ 100 mL	Palm olein, soy oil, coconut oil, high oleic sunflower oil	DHA=11.5 mg/ 100 mL ARA=23 mg/ 100 mL	$31.89 680 g

Note: The above information can change in a matter of months, so research every product carefully. Prices may vary depending on place of purchase.

6

BABY POO
Knowing Their "Business"

Believe it or not, baby's poo is a hot topic among parents. Although some parents are embarrassed to talk about poo, it gives you a sneak peek into what's going on inside baby's little body. Bowel movements should be a daily occurrence, and although changing diapers isn't much fun, those baby poos are vital for a healthy body.

The first poo is the dark, sticky, and tarlike meconium that baby passes soon after birth. It's a mixture of a buildup of skin cells, mucus, amniotic fluid, bile from the gall bladder, and water. Nothing has actually been ingested yet, so it's bacteria-free and almost sterile. Meconium should be completely passed by the end of the third day postpartum.

Once the meconium has cleared, the poo becomes mustard yellow in colour, and the texture is quite liquid with seedy white bits. Breast milk poo is unique in consistency as well as colour because the majority of bacteria in breastfed babies' tummies are *Bifidobacteria*. If your baby drinks formula or has started eating solid food, the stools will be more formed and brown or tan due to the change in the balance of intestinal bacteria away from predominantly *Bifidobacteria*.

Getting the Sticky Stuff Off

Rub an oil such as olive or grape seed on to your newborn's clean bum so that the meconium later wipes off easily.

According to Dr. Nigel Plummer, a prominent microbiologist from the United Kingdom, only 22 percent of the fecal matter from a formula-fed baby will contain *Bifidobacteria* (good bacteria), with the remaining 70 percent containing the undesirable bacteria. In comparison, a breastfed baby's poo contains 95 percent *Bifidobacteria*. We want to encourage the colonization of the good bacteria to help support baby's immune system and digestive function, with the hope of reducing the chance of allergies and improving overall health. To foster the growth of beneficial bacteria, I recommend that all formula-fed babies supplement with a probiotic containing human strains of both *Bifidobacterium infantis* and *Lactobacillus acidophilus* at a level of at least three billion total bacteria per day.

FREQUENCY OF BOWEL MOVEMENTS

TYPICAL BREAST MILK POO

Breastfed babies can have bowel movements anywhere from one to six times a day. And on occasion, your baby may not poo for five days. Breastfed babies use most of what is in their milk, so sometimes, during a growth spurt or around six months when they are almost ready to start solids, there may not be much to eliminate and so you won't see a bowel movement for a few days. This is common and not a huge concern. If your baby hasn't pooed for a week, discuss this with your doctor just to be sure all is well.

Breast milk poo doesn't have a particularly offensive odour—a slightly acidic smell is normal. The consistency is liquid, and it should always be mustard yellow. If it ever has a greenish tinge to it, your baby either isn't getting the hind milk (the fattier breast milk toward the end of a feeding) or has an infection. If it's the former, your baby might be fussier than usual. The fore milk (from the first few minutes of nursing) is more carbohydrate rich and doesn't have the more sustaining fat to keep babies going longer. It's a bit like eating a plain cracker—it doesn't satisfy you until you top it with fat-rich avocado or almond butter. If you see the green poo, try to nurse for as long as possible on one breast and then switch to the other. If your baby is the on-and-off type, keep offering the same breast for that feeding. If the stools are still green, see your doctor to ensure your baby doesn't have an infection. (See "Constipation," below, for tips if your baby isn't pooing frequently.)

TYPICAL FORMULA POO

A formula-fed baby should be pooing at least once a day. Because bacteria in the digestive system of a formula-fed baby are more similar to those in an adult or in a baby who's started on solids, the poo will be similar in consistency, colour, and smell to adult stool. However, it shouldn't be formed or hard. The consistency should be like soft ice cream, and you'll need a few wipes to see a clean bum. Sometimes the stool reflects the smell of the formula. If your baby's poo is particularly offensive-smelling, lingering after you leave the change table, there may be more unfriendly bacteria than good guys present in the digestive tract.

I always recommend giving babies probiotics containing *Bifidobacterium infantis* and *Lactobacillus acidophilus* to help balance the bacteria in the intestines with a better ratio of good to bad guys. Probiotics may also solve any issues with gassiness and lessen the potential for allergies, especially as dairy (most formula is dairy based) is the top allergy in infants and children. Iron absorption from formula is helped by good bacteria keeping the bad bugs that thrive on iron at bay.

DIARRHEA: WATERY POO

Diarrhea happens when the time it takes for food to travel from mouth to toilet or diaper is too fast and so the digestion process can't complete its task of breaking down food particles into nutrients and absorbing water from the intestines. Diarrhea can be serious in an infant because of the potential for dehydration. The wateriness of diarrhea results from the fast transit time, which doesn't allow for reabsorption of water from the intestines. Water reabsorption in the intestines helps to balance hydration in our bodies. This water loss must be replaced orally in order to stay hydrated.

Diarrhea is commonly a symptom of the body trying to get rid of a bacteria, virus, or parasite from something that's either been ingested or passed from another person. Don't try to suppress it too quickly, but rather let the body try to rid itself of what it needs to. Newborns experiencing diarrhea should be seen immediately by a doctor, and the same applies to an infant or child having diarrhea for more than 24 hours. Diarrhea is also common during teething, when it's particularly acidic to a little bum. If diarrhea lasts for a long time and doesn't seem to be related to a virus or bacteria from food contamination, it may be a sign of food sensitivity. There are a few common culprits, including dairy and wheat (see Chapter 7). The only way to treat chronic or long-term diarrhea or even loose stools is to dig until you find the cause. Your doctor might do stool tests to see whether the cause is bacterial or even a parasite, or you may need to remove suspected foods from your diet if breastfeeding, think about changing formula if it has added DHA, or figure out if the source is a food, if your baby's on solids.

Keeping your baby hydrated is essential. If your baby has started solids, expect him to refuse food during an episode of diarrhea, whether the cause is bacterial, viral, or teething. It's better for his body to clear what it needs to before filling back up on food. Do keep up his breast milk or formula intake to ensure he's getting some nutrition. It can take up to two weeks after sickness, especially a gastrointestinal type, for the appetite to go back to normal. I always recommended that parents give acidophilus to recolonize the intestines with good bacteria; in my experience, it has also helped return the appetite to what it was, faster.

No matter what the cause of diarrhea, remove all dairy products from the diet. Milk and dairy products, as well as most formulas, contain a sugar called lactose. When diarrhea hits, the fast transit time clears not only any fibre, food, bacteria, and water from the intestines, but also the lactase enzymes, which digest lactose. With that enzyme missing, the body is unable to digest lactose in dairy products, especially milk or formula, which can lead to instant lactose intolerance, the inability to digest lactose. Lactose intolerance is more common in adults—usually it affects babies only in this situation or in very rare cases. Switch

> ### Other Reasons for Diarrhea
>
> For Breastfed Babies: Because what you eat passes to your baby through breast milk, some possible causes of diarrhea in your diet include getting too much vitamin C or magnesium from a supplement; using antacids containing magnesium salts; eating foods with sorbitol, manitol, and xylitol; consuming milk or other dairy products; and eating spicy food.
>
> For Formula-Fed Babies: There seems to be a correlation between the DHA added to formula and diarrhea in some babies. If your baby is drinking one of these formulas, switch to one without DHA (see Chapter 5 for suggestions), or if you've just started your baby on a new formula (with or without DHA), try a hydrolyzed or lactose-free formula.

to a lactose-free formula (see the table on page 97) for at least two weeks after the diarrhea passes to allow the lactase to build up again and let the intestines heal. If you start back on a lactose formula too early, gassiness or abdominal discomfort may occur.

If your baby was on solid food before the diarrhea, ease slowly back into the regular diet, offering simple foods such as applesauce, mashed banana, puréed vegetables, and wholegrain brown rice or potatoes. Don't start on anything new until bowel movements have gone back to normal. Avoid fatty foods and too much protein, as they are harder to digest and the intestines still need to recover.

Probiotics may lessen the severity and length of diarrhea as they put the good bacteria back into the intestines, where they recolonize and heal the intestinal lining. Homeopathic remedies are often quick to resolve a situation of diarrhea, and some herbal teas, such as peppermint, can be soothing to the digestive tract. Pedialyte and similar rehydrating solutions contain sugar, salt, and water in a specific balance for maximum rehydration. Be careful to avoid sugars from other drinks or food sources, as they can make the diarrhea worse.

TRAVELLER'S DIARRHEA

Travel, whether to Mexico, India, or another province or town, can expose your baby to foreign or unfriendly bacteria. When travelling, it's hard to know where the water comes from that's used for drinking, brushing your teeth, and washing fruits and vegetables in a restaurant. Protecting everyone in the family with probiotics, once again, can help avoid any digestive upsets while you're away from home. Start taking or giving higher doses at least a week before your travel date, and take your supplement with you, continuing the higher dose the entire length of your vacation. On your return, go back to your normal intake.

CONSTIPATION: HARD POO

Constipation, a lack of or incomplete bowel movement, is unfortunately a common problem with infants and children. It includes straining to poo, eliminating a hard or formed stool, as well as passing infrequent or incomplete stool. Again, this situation can be quite different for breastfed and formula-fed babies.

Breastfed Babies

Constipation doesn't usually occur in breastfed babies. A lack of a daily bowel movement is common but is not to be confused with constipation because when breastfed babies do poo, it's not hard and formed. In the early days, your newborn should be having two to three bowel movements a day, sometimes more. If 24 hours go by without a poo, seek help from the breastfeeding clinic or a lactation consultant as your baby may not be getting enough milk as a result of an improper latch (not because you're not producing enough milk).

Breastfed babies can have between one and five poos a day. There doesn't seem to be any particular reason for having more or less. After two to three weeks of age, your baby may start skipping bowel movements for a day or two but continues to be happy and healthy and to gain weight. This is normal. Breast milk is so absorbable and so highly utilized in the body that there may not be as much to eliminate. I've heard of babies going without a poo for a week or two, and in one case, almost a month. Although Canadian breastfeeding expert Dr. Jack Newman doesn't consider this a problem, I'm not convinced. The muscles in the digestive tract (mainly the intestines) perform peristalsis, a process in which said muscles contract to move food through the digestive system. This is a new and important skill for your baby's digestive system to develop. My main concern is that the intestinal muscles may not be developing as they should and become lazy in their function. I've always been of the opinion that regular bowel movements are incredibly important for good health, and this is no exception.

If you've had a few days or more of super-fast diaper changes (with no poo to clean) and your baby is content and shows no fussiness, gas, or pulling her legs up to her belly you don't need to be overly concerned until that changes. Sometimes grunting or straining to have a poo doesn't produce results. If this is the case, you can help by putting your baby to the breast because as the milk goes into the stomach, it stimulates the digestive system lower down to start contracting and moving fecal matter along and out of the body. If that doesn't help, you might try to stimulate the anus, most commonly with a thermometer or well-oiled Q-tip. This should produce results immediately or soon after. Don't allow this to become regular practice, though, as there could be issues behind the constipation that need to be looked into.

When you've been waiting for a bowel movement for a few days or more and it finally vacates the bowel, be prepared for an explosion that can burst right out of the diaper and up baby's back—I've even seen it get in babies' hair. Unfortunately, as Murphy's Law dictates, this never happens at home, where you could simply wash baby from head to toe. No, it happens in the car seat when you're on your way somewhere, *late,* are down to your last wipe, and have no extra clothes. Be sure your diaper bag is well stocked while you're waiting for that poo!

If your baby is having regular problems with infrequent bowel movements, look at what you're eating or drinking in case this is a reaction to a food or drink in the breast milk. See "Baby's Reactions to Breast Milk" in Chapter 4.

FORMULA-FED BABIES

Constipation in a formula-fed baby, unfortunately, is common. It occurs as a reaction either to ingredients in the formula or to the increased concentration of nutrients, minerals, and different fats, particularly palm olein oil.[60] Breast milk contains more water and nutrients and thus needs less digestion than formula. Unlike a breastfeeding baby, a formula-fed baby should poo every day. The consistency of the stool will be unlike that of breastfed babies because of the different bacteria present in the intestines. If your baby becomes constipated on a new formula or while weaning on to formula, I'd suggest looking for an alternative. Parents often wonder whether the iron fortification in the formula causes constipation, but studies show that it's not likely the culprit. Palm olein oil is used as a fatty acid source in most formulas and has been demonstrated to increase constipation in babies.[61] Check the label on your can, or refer to the table on page 92, to see whether your formula contains palm olein oil. (Some labels say "or palm olein oil" because they switch between two oils depending on availability.) I came across only two companies that manufacture formula without it. If the problem still occurs, switch formulas again until

> ### Survey Says ... Reactions from Formula
>
> Results from my online survey showed that 50 percent of moms said their baby had constipation upon starting formula, 2 percent reported skin rash, 4 percent saw diarrhea, and 25 percent reported colic or gassiness and spitting up.[62]

your baby is pooing every day. Consult with your doctor, as well; he might suggest an ultrasound or another treatment.

STARTING SOLIDS = CONSTIPATION?

Constipation in babies who are eating solids can be more common when they start on cereals. Any of the cereals have the potential to cause constipation, but I see it more with rice cereal. The reason for the constipation could be babies' limited starch-digesting enzymes in their digestive systems or the cereal's iron fortification. Although iron in cereal has a fairly good absorption rate (about 5 to 10 percent is absorbed), the form of iron in cereals is often associated with constipation. If your baby has constipation from eating infant cereals, remove the cereal until bowel movements are back to normal, and when reintroducing, offer only small quantities and perhaps switch to another cereal. I've seen babies do well on oatmeal after they've been constipated with rice cereal, but not all will.

As you progress with solids and introduce new foods, constipation may occur because not enough water was added to vegetable purées. Sweet potato, especially, is so fibrous that it needs a lot of water to help that fibre move through the digestive tract. Parsnips also need plenty of water added to the purée.

An overall lack of fibre, water, or both can lead to constipation in anyone, young or old. Meat is a protein-rich food but is lacking in fibre. If you're giving meat to your baby or toddler for added iron and protein in her diet, remember to serve it with fibre-rich vegetables.

I mentioned above that exclusively breastfed babies don't generally suffer from constipation, but this rule changes after solids are introduced. If it's not the food that you're giving to your baby that's causing the constipation, look at your own diet. Foods that often trigger constipation in baby include dairy, wheat, sugar, chocolate, coffee, and gluten (found in wheat, rye, barley, spelt, kamut, and some oats). The only way to find out which food may be causing the constipation is by eliminating some of these possible triggers or any other suspect foods. After avoiding the questionable foods for at least two weeks (four weeks for a more definitive answer), start eating them again. If there's a reaction (remember, it could take three to five days for it to show up), avoid that food and delay introducing it to your baby.

Wheat is a very common food sensitivity that's known to cause constipation. It's high in gluten and can irritate the lining of the intestines. I caution against giving wheat to babies and even toddlers until about 18 months of age. Wheat is a frequently consumed grain that seems to sneak into just about everything. Parents giving toast, cookies, pasta, bagels, or muffins to their babies or toddlers need to keep in mind that all these foods contain wheat and so it can end up being eaten many times throughout the day. The quantity of wheat eaten easily increases as new foods are introduced, especially prepackaged foods of all kinds.

My Story

My second daughter suffered with recurrent constipation from 10 months of age. She was breastfed and eating only fruits, vegetables, beans, and pulses. My diet was fairly restricted already, with no wheat, dairy, and for the most part, sugar. On any occasion that I ate sugar or, worse, chocolate, she'd become constipated, leading to severe pain and crying while trying to poo. Once again, I felt like the worst mother for having eaten something that could cause her that much pain. As soon as I cut sugar out completely, she had regular poos, as I would have expected from such a fibre-rich diet.

Dairy is also associated with constipation, and intake should be evaluated if symptoms appear. Milk, cheese, and yogurt are favourites of both children and adults and, like wheat, make up a large part of our daily intake. Remove them completely for at least two weeks and then reintroduce to see if the same reaction appears. If it does, then once again, keep them out of your diet and go slowly when introducing them directly to your baby. You can replace dairy with other calcium-rich foods, such as green leafy vegetables, amaranth (see the recipe on page 257), almonds, sesame seeds and tahini, organic soy, navy beans, and blackstrap molasses.

SIMPLE, EFFECTIVE TREATMENTS

First, any situation of prolonged constipation should be investigated by your doctor. A common medical treatment is to give mineral oil or use suppositories. Neither is pleasant for anyone. Below are some suggestions to help pass the impacted stool and to make your child more comfortable while you investigate why the constipation is there in the first place.

- Write a food diary of all foods eaten for five days—this should raise some red flags for foods that are regularly eaten and may cause constipation. Remove those foods from mom's diet or the child's diet until the situation resolves.

- Give water to your baby from about nine months of age (or sometimes earlier) as the diet increases in complexity and different fibres are introduced. It can be offered earlier, but may not be successful until your baby gets the hang of the sippy cup. Offering 30 to 60 mL (2 to 4 oz) of water at regular intervals throughout the day should help a constipated baby. Get her to drink as much of it as possible; any water is better than none.

- Give flax seed oil as a stool softener. Doctors offer mineral oil to ease constipation, but if you're giving an oil to soften the stool, your baby might as well get some nutritional benefit from it. Flax seed oil offers both omega-3 and omega-6 essential fatty acids. First offer one teaspoon, increasing to two tablespoons if necessary. But don't become dependent on it—use only as necessary while you figure out the root cause of the constipation.

- Give probiotics to your baby daily. They are very helpful in alleviating constipation by normalizing digestive function. Give an HMF (human microflora by Genestra) product that contains both *Bifidobacterium* and *Lactobacillus* strains of beneficial bacteria. Give three billion bacteria (read the label to see how much is in your product) daily after "milk" or food (*Bifidobacteria infantis* should also be on the label, as it's a specific strain of good bacteria for babies under age one).

- Remove food altogether. If your baby has just started solids and isn't yet eating three regular meals a day, remove the food from his diet and go back to breast milk or formula until you see regular bowel movements. When you start to introduce food once again, start very slowly and only with foods that you know are on the safe list.

- Avoid sugar completely. You might have to look at your diet if breastfeeding, and if you consume a lot of sugar, avoid it as much as you can. Try dried fruit as a sweet alternative.

- If formula-feeding, be sure that the formula isn't "extra iron" fortified or contains palm olein oil (known to cause constipation and other digestive issues). See Chapter 5 for more suggestions.

- Give your baby dried fruits. Prunes, dried apricots, and raisins all have a laxative effect and can be given to clear the blockage. But don't rely on prune purée or prune juice for a daily bowel movement—this treats the symptom but doesn't get to the cause of the problem.

- Apply castor oil to your baby's abdomen to help clear the blockage. Rub a loonie-sized amount over the abdomen and lower back before bed. Put on the

From the Mouths of Moms

"Liam had been constipated since he started on solids at six months. I gave him just fruit and vegetables—pears, banana, avocado, sweet potato, carrots, beans, and prunes—but despite a voracious appetite (and water after), he never had a painless poo following solids. I took him to the doctor twice after he screamed in agony trying to go, and they prescribed lactulose indefinitely, as well as suppositories. They recommended more fibre and continuing to feed solids and said that his body would learn to process the food at some point. However, I can't believe this is normal—I hate the medicine, the crying—it's not right! Liam was given antibiotics at one month of age. When he was a newborn, he used to have over 10 very gassy, explosive poos a day. So I stopped all dairy, and within a day or two, he was down to only 1 poo a day."

My recommendation to mom was stop all solid food and breastfeed until the constipation cleared and he had painless bowel movements. I also advised giving Liam HMF Natogen (infant probiotics) daily. I also asked mom to remove all dairy once again, try to eliminate wheat, and watch her intake of sugar, as it might be feeding any candida living in his gut.

Mom emailed a few days later, once his poo had gone back to typical breast milk poo and he was having painless bowel movements. She thought he was ready to try solids again. She reintroduced one meal a day of butternut squash, and he didn't poo for three days. I then suggested castor oil be rubbed on his abdomen every night before bed and one teaspoon of flax seed oil be given as well. Mom reported that he was pooing again. She moved on to pears, slowly, once a day, and then I got this report: "Your advice completely turned things around, and Liam went from gasping in pain and wailing trying to go poo to a happy little boy who poos a few times a day without any trouble! I was careful to just give him small portions for the first month, just once a day, and he now eats purée twice a day!" Mom continues to watch her diet and supplement with HMF Natogen. At last report, Liam had some constipation again, but mom is doing a great job of managing it while looking out for the cause.

diaper as usual and older onesies or pyjamas, as the oil may get on them (though it does wash out).

- Consider osteopathy, a hands-on, noninvasive treatment safe for day-old babies and older, which may help by making sure that nerves associated with muscle contraction within the digestive system aren't restricted or constricted. I've seen many babies treated by an osteopath return to normal bowel function. It's a simple therapy that all babies should have at some point in their lives, if not a few times a year.

All the above recommendations are meant only to help ease the situation. You still need to be a good detective and find the reason why your baby is constipated in the first place. Treating the symptom does not solve the problem and can lead to fear of pooing, even in babies. Hard, compacted stools are not only painful, but can cause tiny fissures in the anus, leading to bleeding and even more pain when trying to poo. That's enough to make any parent willing to do whatever it takes to avoid the problem. Hey, I gave up chocolate and sugar (definitely not easy when I was getting fast energy hits from sugar), and if I can do it, you can too!

GASSY TUMMY AND BABY TOOTS

Gassiness is a common condition that often causes a lot of pain. Some babies tell you about the pain by crying, and at times they can be inconsolable. It seems that some babies are born gassy and others develop gassiness with the introduction of solid food. Whatever the age, there could be many reasons for it.

NEWBORN GAS

Gassiness in newborns up to the age of three months is sometimes referred to as colic or fussiness. The persistent crying for, it seems, no particular reason is exhausting for new parents and babies. Whether you have a diagnosis of colic or not, the reasons behind gassiness are possibly the same.

Your baby may be reacting to something in your diet if you're breastfeeding. Trial-and-error elimination is the only way to find out for sure—dairy, wheat, chocolate, coffee, garlic, spices, cabbage, broccoli, and cauliflower might be good places to start. Dairy is the most common offender, with wheat and chocolate a close second. Eliminate what you suspect for at least two weeks before reintroducing. Some babies take longer to show an improvement.

Your baby may be reacting to his formula. Try to pinpoint when the problem started, and if it started with formula or with increased intake, consider changing formulas. Some babies might be fine on 120 mL (4 oz) of formula, but as that level increases, symptoms appear. See Chapter 5 for suggestions.

> ### Sweeping Statements
>
> My two-month-old was extremely fussy at 6 p.m. every day, and a friend asked if I was eating chocolate—she thought this might be the cause. I stopped eating chocolate, and the fussiness disappeared.
> —DIANE, MOM OF THREE

The flow of breast milk or formula might be too fast. Swallowing air along with milk causes more air to get into the stomach and either come back up the way it went in or become trapped lower in the digestive tract. Burp your baby throughout her feeding if possible to release air. Also, position your baby so that while nursing her head is higher than the nipple (hard to imagine, I know, but try a football hold and then lean back into a chair while supporting the back of the head). This should slow down the flow into baby's mouth. Make your baby work for the flow instead of trying to keep up with both gravity and breast milk flow.

In formula-fed babies, buy bottles that help eliminate extra air or have fewer holes in the nipple to reduce the flow. Also, look at the ingredients in your formula and perhaps switch to one that isn't sweetened with corn syrup or sucrose. These two sweeteners might be feeding any bad bacteria present, which give off gas and increase discomfort (see Chapter 5).

Your baby might be getting too much fore milk versus hind milk. Fore milk is the first breast milk in your baby's meal. It's high in lactose and water, whereas the hind milk supplies fat to sustain your baby. Too much fore milk without the hind milk can make a baby gassy and fussy. To ensure that baby gets more hind milk, try to completely drain the milk by compressing your breast once your baby slows down nursing toward the end of feeding on one side.

If you were exposed to antibiotics during pregnancy, labour, and delivery or while breastfeeding, there may be a higher percentage of unfriendly bacteria to good guys in her digestive tract. Probiotics are a safe and effective treatment of gassiness and other abdominal symptoms and should be given to baby as soon as possible (see the Resources for details on HMF Natogen).

STINKY TOOTS AND POO

Most toots and poo don't smell of roses, but they certainly shouldn't leave a lingering aroma that sends everyone for cover. The smell of your baby's poo will reflect what he's drinking or eating. If it's sweet potato, it will have a sweet smell and orange colour. In cases of really stinky toots or poo, you can suspect that there are less desirable bacteria present in the digestive tract. Along with the unfriendly bacteria might be food that isn't being digested or broken down properly, which increases the nose-holding aroma. You may not realize how sweet-smelling your nursery can be until you squash the bad bacteria by having them fight it out with good bacteria, or probiotics. After a few days of taking probiotics, baby's digestive and immune systems will be functioning better, making him happier, and leaving the person changing his diaper to breathe much easier.

INEFFICIENT BURPING OR TOOTING

Some babies have a hard time dispelling gas from either end. Patiently burping your baby by supporting the front of her body on your chest and slightly over your shoulder and rubbing in an upward motion should help. Some babies do well with the pat style of burping, so try both to see which is more effective. A football hold, with her belly down along your forearm, head (or cheek, actually) in your hand, and legs straddling the inside of your elbow, is often a comfortable position. Pressure on the abdominal area from either the forearm or even abdominal massage often helps to alleviate gas and discomfort.

SUPPORTIVE RELIEF

Osteopathy is a hands-on treatment that aims to release restriction and constriction gently so that normal function can resume.[63] Osteopaths perform craniosacral therapy within their treatments that can help alleviate any tension between the cranium and sacrum and associated nerves or organs. For the treatment of gassiness, colic, constipation—well, anything really—osteopathy can be amazingly effective. Tema Stein, a Toronto-based pediatric osteopath, explains that certain situations while in utero or during delivery (the birth itself or use of vacuum or forceps, for example) can lead to health effects later: "If there has been any squeezing of the cranium (skull), you are squeezing on the contents (the nerves and brain). Depending on where the squeezing happens, it can affect different aspects of health, such as gassiness, constipation, colic, ear infections, poor latch, strong gag reflex to name a few."[64] Homeopathic remedies also can be very useful in situations of colic. If you're unfamiliar with homeopathy or don't know a homeopath, look for combinations of the most common remedies for colic, such as Boiron's Cocyntal. They're safe to give to mom and baby and are incredibly effective once you find the remedy that best matches the symptoms. They're available at most pharmacies and health food stores. Otherwise, consult with a naturopath or homeopath for specific remedies.

Gripe water also helps with gassiness or colic. But most gripe water is usually a mixture of sugar and water, and I'd recommend staying away from any product containing sugar for your baby. A herbal, sugar-free gripe water, such as Colic Calm (containing fennel), is a better alternative. Read the label before giving anything to your baby.

Fennel oil has shown great results for reducing colic in babies. In a 2003 study, 121 infants with colic were given either a placebo or an emulsion of fennel seed oil.[65] Colic symptoms decreased a whopping 45 percent in the infants taking the fennel seed oil formula, compared with only a 5 percent reduction in symptoms in those taking the placebo formula. Fennel seems to "reduce intestinal spasm and to increase the movement (motility) of the small intestines," two factors often contributing to the development of colic.[66]

Beneficial bacteria may be lacking in the case of any gassiness, not just with colic-type symptoms. Good bacteria do great things like produce vitamins, digest the sugar in milk, and maintain acidity in the intestines to keep bad bacteria under control. When a baby is first born, she has a higher

How Much Bacteria?

Ten times more bacteria are present in our intestines than anywhere else in our bodies. And in the intestines, there are about 500 types of bacteria, a lot of them not fully understood by even the best researchers.

level of *Lactobacillus* bacteria in the intestines, which changes within the first week to primarily *Bifidobacterium*, especially in the breastfed baby. If your baby was born by Caesarean section or has been introduced to formula, that balance can be altered, perhaps not for the better, so give probiotics to your baby daily.

Doctors have begun recommending a pharmaceutical brand of probiotics for the treatment of colic research that showed positive results. This is a hopeful development for new parents who don't consult a naturopath or nutritionist—the usual way to find out about probiotics.

Probiotics support the development of the digestive system and so can help in many ways (let's not forget the significant decrease they bring to the potential for allergies). There are no side effects to giving probiotics.[67] Ensure that your infant probiotics supplement includes *Bifidobacterium infantis* as well as *Lactobacillus* strains of bacteria at a level of approximately three billion. It should be given after nursing or formula-feeding one to two times a day, depending on the severity and history of your baby's symptoms of gas, constipation, or diarrhea. A breastfeeding mom can also take an adult probiotic supplement to enhance her immune system; even though the probiotics that mom takes don't reach breast milk, she'll pass on immune factors that get into the breast milk and support the baby's immune system further.

7

ALLERGY AND THE IMMUNE SYSTEM

Allergies, especially in relation to food, are being called a modern epidemic. It's a scary prospect to have a child with an allergy that has no "cure." The terms *allergy, food intolerance, sensitivity,* and *hypersensitivity* are all used to describe reactions to food and can describe the same symptoms, leading to misunderstanding and confusion. Making sense of it all isn't an easy task. There are many theories, opinions, and hypotheses about what is causing the rapidly increasing incidence of allergies. Health Canada reported in 2007 that "current estimates are that food allergies affect as many as 6% of young children and 3% to 4% of adults."[68] I'd suggest that those numbers are rapidly increasing.

To help you understand the differences between all of this jargon, I'll first explain the immune system and how it works and develops in your baby. Later in the chapter I'll give you suggestions on how to reduce the risk of allergy and some possible ways to manage allergies and food sensitivities. Numerous books have been written about allergies and food sensitivity, so for far more in-depth analysis and detail than I can put in this book (otherwise, it would be a book on allergy), refer to the Resources for further reading.

For a bit of clarity, a food allergy involves the immune system, and the response is usually more severe than with a food intolerance or sensitivity. Reactions or symptoms of either allergy or sensitivity can be anywhere from uncomfortable (in the case of gas from wheat or dairy intolerance) to life-threatening (as with peanut allergy and anaphylactic shock), and anything in between. I'll discuss both situations later in the chapter.

OUR PROTECTOR: THE IMMUNE SYSTEM

The immune system works 24/7 to keep us healthy. We are exposed daily to bacteria and viruses, which, for the most part, are neutralized by the immune system. Days, weeks, or months can go by with us being totally unaware that the immune system's doing its job until one day we get sick with a cold, flu, diarrhea, or vomiting. It's then suddenly apparent that the immune system has failed to neutralize a bacterium or virus or maybe even a parasite, leading to the illness.

Our immune system usually doesn't attack our organs, tissues, or cells (this doesn't hold true in the case of autoimmune disorders). The normal cells, tissues, and organs in our bodies, which we might call our "safe residents" or the "self" (meaning what is a part of our self), are covered in a protein that the immune system recognizes, so it leaves them alone to go about their business. Just about everything else—dead tissue, foreign invaders, or anything that the immune system doesn't recognize or that doesn't have this protective, recognizable coating—is attacked, neutralized, and eaten up by immune cells called *phagocytes* or *neutrophils*. Believe it or not, your immune system adapts during pregnancy so that your baby, a foreign being, can grow inside you. So as not to reject mom, your baby doesn't fully develop its immune system before birth (the immune system stays immature for a while after birth, too). Your body's ability to "down-regulate" the immune system to host your baby during gestation is a remarkable adaptation. Many women who suffer from allergies or sensitivities to food remark that while pregnant, they can enjoy foods that they couldn't before pregnancy. I've known someone with celiac disease (an allergy to gluten) who was able to eat wheat and other gluten-containing grains throughout her pregnancy without the usual reactions. It's also common for colds and flus to linger during pregnancy, further demonstrating how the immune system becomes more tolerant, or down-regulates, during pregnancy.

THE IMMUNE ARMY

The immune system can be thought of as an army of generals, soldiers, killers, and clean-up crew. It's helpful to know how each part of the army acts in our bodies to better understand why an allergic reaction happens.

Immune Cells

White blood cells (also called leukocytes) are known as the main defenders of the immune system. White blood cells include:

- Lymphocytes—the generals. They travel around the blood and lymph system looking for any invaders they don't recognize and mount an attack with the help of others. There are two types of lymphocytes—B and T lymphocytes. Both are developed from stem cells in the liver and bone marrow. T lymphocytes mature and are under the instruction of the thymus gland (part of the immune system), found behind the breastbone. In the family of T lymphocytes there are T-helper cells (TH cells), T suppressor cells, and natural killer cells (NK cells). The TH cells help to activate the B lymphocytes to produce antibodies (immunoglobulins, or Igs—see below), while the T suppressor cells turn off the activation once the invader has been dealt with and hold up the victory flag. NK cells are like germ warfare—they produce toxins that can annihilate anything foreign. Both B and T cells leave behind memory cells so that if the same antigen (perceived foreign invader) crosses their path again, they will mount an attack and do it all over again but more quickly and efficiently.
- Monocytes (found in blood) and macrophages (found in tissues)—the clean-up crew. These cells finish off and clean up what the others started by engulfing and digesting the invader through inflammation and signalling other troops that there's a war going on. Monocytes present the invader to the T cells so that they can recognize more of their kind in the body and continue the attack. (That's what I call teamwork!)
- Granulocytes—the soldiers. These make up the majority of the white blood cells and include neutrophils, cosinophils, and basophils. They also help the clean-up crew and engulf invaders, damaged cells, or debris, supporting the monocytes and macrophages.
- Mast cells—the front line of defence. These are mainly residential cells that are found close to entranceways into the body, for example, the mouth and eyes. They produce histamine, which most of us are familiar with. It creates itching, redness, inflammation, and flushing in an allergic response.

The main points of entry of any foreign particle can be through the skin (topically or injected), via the mouth or eyes, up the nose, inhaled into the lungs, or even passed up into the urethra. All of our epithelial cells (or internal skin), at each of these entry points, are coated with mucus to slow down or stop the invader in its tracks. The eyes defend with both mucus and tears, which contain an enzyme called lysozyme that breaks down the cell walls of many bacteria. Saliva is alkaline and antibacterial. The nasal passages and lungs are coated in mucus and trap invaders in the mucus, which are then blown out, sniffed or coughed up, and swallowed (sorry, not a nice picture, but it happens). Mast cells also line the nasal passages, throat, lungs, and skin. Any bacteria or virus that wants to gain entry to your body must first make it past these defences.

THE IMMATURE ARMY

When your baby is born his immune system is not mature, meaning that it has a lot of learning to do. It can take about two years for your baby's immune system to fully mature and become an effective army of immune cells working together to fight off foreign invaders.

The Five Classes of Antibodies Called Immunoglobulins (Igs)

- IgE—involved in type 1 allergic reactions. The presence of this antibody is a marker for an allergy that your doctor might test for with a scratch test.
- IgG—the most abundant, making up 75 percent of all antibodies in the body. These antibodies are passed on to the fetus through the placenta and are found in breast milk, along with IgA. IgG attacks bacteria, viruses, and fungi by neutralizing and destroying them. It's also thought to be involved in approximately 60 percent of allergic reactions and is more commonly associated with food sensitivity.
- IgA—found in breast milk, saliva, sweat, tears, blood, the lungs, and intestinal mucosa. It's also known as secretory IgA, or sIgA. It protects against foreign invaders before they can enter the body. IgA is most abundant in the digestive system. A deficiency of IgA is an indicator of allergy, because it gets used up in calming the allergic reaction.
- IgM—one of the largest. This front-liner operating in the bloodstream only comes out strong at the beginning of an infection to disable bacteria. It doesn't cross the placenta.
- IgD—makes up a very small percentage of the immunoglobulin team. It signals the spleen (another immune organ) that the B cells are ready for action.

In the beginning, your baby relies on the immunity she took from you through the placenta while in utero, on the way out in the birth canal, and in colostrum first and then breast milk, two to three days after birth. This is one important reason for exclusively breastfeeding your baby, even if just for a short while. If possible, avoid supplementing with formula either in the hospital or after you've come home—formula doesn't provide antibodies or immune support, and it is a potential allergen.

The immune system takes time to mature and strengthen as it practises recognizing what is foreign, or "non-self," while ignoring "self." The more it gets to flex its muscles by mounting an attack and winning the battle, the stronger the army becomes. And although it might seem as if your baby has a constantly runny nose (this may also be due to a food intolerance or allergy), his immunoglobulins, neutrophils, mast cells, and lymphocytes are learning what to do with different attackers. But if the immune system does not get the chance to develop in the way it needs to—perhaps a certain aspect isn't challenged and doesn't develop properly—something may go awry. Hyperresponse, or an army overreacting to something that's not a foreign invader, such as dairy, might lead to the perpetual runny nose as the immune system keeps on producing mucus to try to capture and eliminate the invader—in this case, dairy.

KEEPING CLEAN—OR NOT?

How do we learn how to do things in life? Something new is presented to us, and through practice we master how to do it. The exact same thing happens in the immune system. It needs practice dealing with foreign invaders, and if it doesn't get the chance to build itself up through practice, it may never reach its full potential. The immune system needs exposure to bacteria, viruses, fungus, and other pathogens (foreign invaders) in order to react and become stronger. These are all things that most parents desperately try to keep their babies safe from as they sanitize everything, including hands, toys, floors, and anything that goes near their mouths and might lead to sickness. But we may actually be doing more harm than good with this practice. I'm not saying that hygiene isn't important, and especially in recent years, with so many potentially harmful situations from superbugs, crazily named flus, and quarantinable illnesses, we want to keep our children from harm. It's understandable. But what if this constant sanitization is contributing to the increased incidence of allergy? Some dirt, germs, viruses, fungi, and other nasties put the immune army through its paces, increasing its strength each time. The more the immune system is confronted, the stronger it gets. Why does your child get a cold or cough? If that's all she gets (as opposed to secondary infections such as chest or ear infections), the immune system is doing its job. A compromised immune system or underfunctioning immune army needs to be assessed along with the history of that child to figure out what may have led to the immune system being unable to attack, defend, and kill illness.

IMMUNITY FROM THE BEGINNING

Babies are "sterile" at birth. When they travel through the birth canal, this is, in a sense, their passageway into the big wide world full of bacteria. Mom's vagina is colonized with beneficial bacteria and possibly some fungus *(Candida albicans)* or unfriendly bacteria, such as strep B, which baby takes on before entering either the hospital room or home, in a home birth. No matter where birth takes place, the beneficial bacteria in the vagina help protect your baby from the billions of bacteria in the world she has just entered. Babies born by Caesarean section don't travel through this passageway, and because they miss this important step, might be lacking in immune protection. There may be an association between Caesarean section birth and higher risk of allergies.

Your baby has taken on your antibodies in utero, including IgE and IgA, for protection as her immune system continues to develop. Nutrients found especially in breast milk supply the immune system with the fuel it needs to function properly. Breast milk contains the antibodies IgE, IgA, and IgM, as well as lactoferrin, which bind to iron in baby's intestines, making it unavailable for bad bacteria to use as fuel. Other immune soldiers are present in breast milk to keep potential bacteria in check. Formula companies have yet to add immunoglobulins or other immune-boosting elements to their products—but one day this might happen.

THE IMMUNE ARMY'S FUEL

Supporting the army is crucial. If it doesn't get adequate nutrition, it's going to be sluggish, fatigued, and unable to rally the troops in defending the body.

Nutrients, including vitamins A, C, E, all the B vitamins including B12 and folic acid, and the minerals zinc and copper, allow the army to function by producing lymphocytes as needed, increasing natural killer cell activity, and producing anti-bodies. Inadequate nutrition would be like sending troops to war while on hunger strike!

The wrong fuel also slows the troops down, and sugar is one of the worst. One teaspoon of sugar can stop the immune complexes for up to eight hours. That's a staggering thought. With other possible causes of immune depression, including pesticides, medical drugs, stress, *Candida albicans,* environmental pol-lution, antibiotic use, trauma, food allergy, and alcohol (not all are applicable for your baby, of course), it's amazing that we fight anything off at all, but somehow we do. However, perhaps our immune system isn't fighting to the best of its abil-ity, which might be the start of a few issues, including allergy.

ANTIBIOTICS: IMMUNE SUPPORT OR NOT?

One of the major medical breakthroughs of our time, antibiotics have saved countless lives in life-threatening situations. Unfortunately, as they've become more commonplace, they're also being overused. Antibiotics are incredibly important in certain situations and may be recommended by your doctor or even your dentist, but they now make up an increasing percentage of prescribed med-icines.

In my years of practising as a nutritionist, I've come across many children who were treated with antibiotics. This is understandable in certain situations; however, so many times I hear that ear infections, for instance, were treated with three, four, or more courses of antibiotics before tubes were put in a child's ears under general anaesthetic. I find this is a mind-boggling method of treatment. After the second prescription of antibiotics, why did no one question why they weren't working? Had a superbug made its way into the ear canal?

Doctors are taught to treat the disease, symptom, or illness. And antibiotics are one treatment they have in their doctor's kit. If one kind doesn't work, maybe another will do the job. I recently heard of a child who was given six different types of antibiotics to treat an ear infection. Unbelievable. I understand the logic, but there must come a point when someone has to say, "STOP!" Take a step back and look at what else might be going on—a food allergy, an immune system not working as it should, or maybe something structural that an osteopath or chiropractor could help with. The negative effects on that child's immune system and digestive system after so many courses of antibiotics may cause more problems than the ear infection. Furthermore, many researchers are still divided as to whether antibiotics are actually effective at all in treating ear infections.

When antibiotics are taken, about one hundred thousand billion beneficial bacteria are destroyed in the intestines. When the course is over, it can take months for them to be replenished. This is an opportunity for fungi, bacteria, and other antibiotic-resistant organisms to proliferate. It's common to see symptoms of diarrhea, gastritis, and fungal infection after antibiotic use, and there's even the potential for more serious bacteria to take a hold, leading to secondary infections (and then more antibiotics). Diarrhea is dangerous for an infant because it can lead to dehydration. And fungal infection, or *Candida albicans,* is an absolute nuisance that can cause many uncomfortable and annoying symptoms of thrush in both mom and baby and also depresses immune function. The immune system then becomes so busy trying to keep the *Candida albicans* or bacteria at bay that it's not as available to fight off the next passerby's sneeze, bringing new bacteria to fight off.

Antibiotics have their place and are sometimes the only way to deal with an illness. However, if they have to be taken, it's essential during and after a course of antibiotics to take probiotics, which have been clinically proven to dramatically reduce negative symptoms, including diarrhea, and lessen the disruption to the beneficial bacterial environment.[69]

Another situation that occurs with antibiotic use is that white blood cell (the general) production is turned off. The antibiotics are doing the job of the immune system, but only up to a

Hindsight: Your History of Antibiotic Use

Think back to pregnancy. Were antibiotics given during your pregnancy? Maybe during labour and delivery for a fever or strep B? Or postnatal while breastfeeding? Was your infant suspected to have an infection or maybe swallowed meconium? Did he have a urinary tract or ear infection? There are so many possibilities for exposure to antibiotics for both mom and baby. Without the active recolonization of the gut with billions of specific good bacteria, both mom and baby are in a weaker immune situation.

point. When the general can't rally his soldiers and clean-up crew, the infection may never be completely dealt with.

Overuse of Antibiotics and Superbugs

Superbug is a word that the father of penicillin, Sir Alexander Fleming, may not have considered when he discovered the first antibiotic. He would have known after further testing that there were some micro-organisms that were resistant to his new find. But since that time, micro-organisms that were killed by antibiotics have mutated into superbugs that can't be treated by antibiotics. On the rise now are serious illnesses from antibiotic-resistant bugs such as *Clostridium difficile* (a diarrhea-causing pathogen), *Staphylococcus aureus* (a bacteria found on the skin and mucous membranes), and many others. The mention of "superbug" brings a feeling of dread, as even the strongest antibiotics are of no use. Studies show that of the most effective treatments for *C. difficile* is probiotics—recolonizing the digestive tract with good bacteria has brought improvement to very sick patients.

HEATING THINGS UP: FEVER

A fever is seen in an increase in body temperature above the normal 37°C (98.6°F). Fever usually comes on as the body's response to a bacterial or viral invasion—viruses usually have a low-grade fever hovering around 38 to 39°C (100.4 to 102.2°F), and bacterial infection is 39°C (102.2°F) and higher. Many viruses and bacteria don't survive in the body with an elevated temperature, and the heating-up increases the production, speed, and effectiveness of all white blood cells.

Complications of a fever include dehydration and febrile seizures—a convulsion in young children, usually lasting a minute or so, that's caused by a sudden spike in their temperature. They may be genetic and occur in a very small percentage of children, usually without long-term negative effects. Medical attention is necessary if your child suffers a seizure.

It's most common to treat a fever with acetaminophen or something similar to make the child more comfortable and to bring down the fever. However, allowing the immune system and its army to deal with this challenge is preferable if possible. Remember that it's in training and needs to flex its muscles to try to win this assault and put up the victory flag. It's important to consult your doctor if a

From the Mouths of Moms

I first met Sophie when she was five months old. Her mom brought her to see me with chronic blood in her poo and digestive discomfort upsetting her sleep. The blood started when Sophie was one week old. During our consultation, mom and I figured out that the bleeding had actually started three days after mom had to take antibiotics for mastitis. That seemed to be the trigger for Sophie's symptoms. Although mom did everything she could to try to modify her diet—she cut out dairy and soy as recommended by her doctor and slowly started to see an improvement—this didn't eliminate the blood altogether. Doctors monitored Sophie as she met all her milestones and her weight climbed without concern. Mom continued to breastfeed and research as much as she could to try to find out what could be going on. To test whether Sophie's problem was related to milk or food intolerance, she also tried giving her regular milk-based formula one day, which she promptly threw up and vomited for the rest of the night. Blood tests showed that Sophie likely had allergic colitis (a difficulty with certain foods that causes parts of the bowel to swell and bleed). Otherwise, her blood tests came back normal, and Sophie took an iron supplement daily (blood loss depletes iron levels). Mom had tried giving Sophie hypoallergenic formula; however, Sophie refused bottle-feeding. Two weeks before I met Sophie, mom had also taken gluten, fish, eggs, nuts, beef, and sesame seeds out of her diet, and that lessened the blood in Sophie's poo.

I gave mom lots of recipes to help her feed herself on a restricted diet and recommended that mom take a very high dose of probiotics, as well as a good multinutrient for breastfeeding moms, and give Sophie HMF Natogen (infant probiotics). Mom noted that Sophie was more unsettled for the first few days of taking the probiotics, but she persevered, and after about three days, Sophie became more comfortable, her sleep improved, and the blood started to lessen slightly. After 10 days, mom wrote that there was no visible blood in Sophie's poo and she was now on full dose of probiotics without discomfort. And as I write this story, Sophie is doing very well—mom's been on her restricted diet for almost six weeks (she has tried almonds, which didn't sit so well with Sophie, and fish without any problems) and both are still taking probiotics—and there's still no blood in her poo. Mom is now gearing up for a very slow introduction of solid food, anticipating that it might take a while and she'll have a few setbacks, but remains hopeful that Sophie will do well with solids.

fever persists, if your child seems listless, or if you're worried about serious illness. But for those times when the temperature is on the rise, let the body learn to do what it needs to do and fight it off. Offering water to sip is important to prevent dehydration, but keep in mind that although you would like your child to eat something, the appetite is usually suppressed in times of illness and fever. Supporting the immune system with vitamin C is a simple yet powerful strategy: Put some vitamin C powder into his water and let him sip it while resting. Lukewarm baths and cold water compresses, or my favourite, cold, wet cotton socks covered by wool or woolly socks (usually adult size) to draw the heat away from the head to the feet, are all effective ways to treat a fever with hydrotherapy (water therapy).

HOLES IN A GARDEN HOSE: LEAKY GUT

Leaky gut may sound like a strange term, but it encompasses the porous state of the intestines perfectly. Ideally, our intestines are a complete entity, with strength in the mucosa, or internal skin, of the intestinal wall. Like a garden hose, cell structure is strong all the way along the length of the small intestine, allowing chewed food particles to enter and stay put while enzymes break them down into smaller molecules, which are transported across the intestinal wall into the bloodstream for use elsewhere in the body. In a large portion of the population, it's as if the garden hose (the intestine) has been attacked by a hole punch, allowing the water that you want to reach your planter to leak out all over the driveway. This, essentially, is what leaky gut looks like. Within the intestines, there are tiny holes (not that you'd be able to see them with the naked eye) that allow some food particles that haven't been digested or broken down yet, as well as bacteria and toxins, to cross into the bloodstream. The circulating immune army is then alerted to these foreign invaders, the food particles. The immune army doesn't differentiate between a nut or dairy particle and bacteria or virus and attacks by producing antibodies. So, in the situation of leaky gut, the immune army is always hard at work defending you against your last meal.

Leaky gut is essential in babies—it's how they survive. The description of an immature digestive system takes into account this leaky gut that all babies are born with. The holes in their intestines allow the minerals, vitamins, antibodies, proteins, carbohydrates, and fats found in breast milk to be easily absorbed and transported into the bloodstream. Formula is partially "digested," or broken down, already to ease the digestion of its ingredients, and formula companies are always doing research to come up with improved absorption and digestion with minimal reactions. While on the subject of formula, perhaps you can now see why some babies commonly react to a dairy formula that hasn't been hydrolyzed, or broken down, as the larger milk protein molecules leak from the intestines into the bloodstream, where they shouldn't be. The immune system comes along, producing antibodies, and an allergy begins. Dairy is one of the most common allergies in infants and children, and this is why. As your baby gets older, the holes get patched up and her digestive system becomes stronger; with less leaky gut, there's less potential for allergies.

> ### Symptoms of Leaky Gut
>
> Just about any symptom can be attributed to leaky gut, but here's a list to fully understand the extent of how it can affect the body: asthma, abdominal pain, indigestion, chronic joint pain, chronic muscle pain, poor immunity, foggy thinking, confusion, gas, mood swings, and nervousness. It also gives rise to poor memory, anxiety, fatigue, recurrent vaginal infections, skin rashes, diarrhea, bedwetting, recurrent bladder infections, constipation, shortness of breath, bloating, aggressive behaviour, and digestive diseases of ulcerative colitis, food allergy and intolerance, and irritable bowel syndrome. Most of this list won't be relevant to your baby, but it illustrates the far-reaching effects of having holes that aren't supposed to be there in the intestines (or garden hose!).

CLASSIC OR TYPE 1 ALLERGY

The term *allergy* refers to a misguided reaction by the immune system to what it perceives as a foreign invader. A nonallergic individual can be challenged by the same "foreign invader," such as a food particle, and not produce a reaction. Allergy was first defined in the mid-1920s to describe an adverse reaction to food in which the immune system is involved by producing IgE antibodies. This definition is still in use within the medical community, but today reactions to foods are far more commonplace and so the symptomatology of allergies may need to be extended from this original definition.

Classical symptoms of allergies can range from a slightly runny nose to anaphylaxis. Other allergic symptoms include coughing, wheezing, itching, swelling of lips, eyes, and/or tongue (anaphylaxis), shortness of breath, itchy mouth, vomiting, diarrhea, headache, and hives and other skin reactions. Allergies also show in situations of autism, celiac disease, colitis and Crohn's disease, eczema, asthma, and migraines. Swelling of the throat or airway needs immediate medical attention.

The immune system can react to dust, mould, pollen, animal hair, insect venom, drugs (such as penicillin and tetracycline), metals (most commonly nickel), food additives, chemicals found in household cleaners, pesticides, and even modern adulterations in GM organisms.

It seems as if the immune system's confused in its reactions. But why and how? These are literally million-dollar questions that parents of allergic children would give their right arm for the answer to. Reacting to peanuts, for instance, seems such a strange thing. A peanut isn't a bacteria, parasite, or virus that can cause illness in the body, so why does the immune system react this way? And why do some people tolerate peanuts while others can die from ingesting microscopic amounts? It all comes back to the individual's immune system.

Researchers are trying desperately to understand the mechanisms of allergy with the hope of eliminating it altogether. I recently attended a conference, "The Development Origins of Disease," given by microbiologist Dr. Nigel Plummer, who's known internationally for his work with both fish oils and probiotics. He had an enlightening way of describing some contributing factors to allergies. Armed with numerous studies to illustrate his point, Dr. Plummer explained how a

Genetically Modified Foods

Genetically modified (GM) foods are a new invention by large companies trying to feed our growing population (and make a buck or two in the process). There are four major GM food crops—soybeans, corn, canola, and cotton. All are used to make vegetable oils, and soy and corn components are used in many processed foods.

GM seeds are resistant to herbicides, allowing the crops to be sprayed without the plant dying from the chemicals. Some see genetic modification to the seed as revolutionizing food today. For most, though, this is tampering with nature and an unpredictable practice.

lack of beneficial microflora (or good bacteria) in a newborn's digestive system doesn't allow for the normal development of a balanced immune system. If you recall, earlier in this chapter I mentioned that a woman's immune system down-regulates during pregnancy so as not to reject the growing fetus, and vice versa. Because of this, baby is born with an immature immune system. The cell-mediated (or TH1) side of his immune system is down-regulated, while his anti-body response (antibody mediated or TH2 side) is dominant. This imbalance means that your baby is born biased toward allergy as his antibodies react to perceived foreign invaders. The balancing these two aspects of the immune system by stimulating the TH1 side starts when your baby takes on your beneficial bacteria during delivery through the nose, mouth, and mucous membranes as he travels through the birth canal. Unfortunately, this important step is missed when babies are born by Caesarean section or antibiotics are given to mom during delivery and even while breastfeeding. But the good news is that you can stimulate and mature the nonallergic TH1 side with infant probiotics, which will help rebalance or steer the immune system away from the TH2 allergic response. I highly recommend supplementing newborn babies with human microflora strains of *Bifidobacterium infantis* and *Lactobacillus acidophilus*. This will help to replace any missed or lessened amount of beneficial bacteria and, ideally, reduce allergic reactions and symptoms such as eczema and asthma (which are IgE antibody responses). The key here seems to be that both mom and baby take probiotics—mom while pregnant and while breastfeeding, and baby as soon as she is born.

Dr. Plummer is involved in a large double-blind, placebo-controlled trial (a long name for a trial where the researchers and the patients don't know who is given the real thing and who is given a placebo) in South Wales, where he and his team are aiming to find out if probiotics could possibly prevent child-onset type 1 or true allergy (IgE). They are using the HMF (human microflora) product including *Bifidobacterium* and *Lactobacillus infantis* and *casei* strains of good bacteria. I've been eagerly awaiting the results, but even though they haven't yet been published, this trial has given more credibility to the use of probiotics, as the HMF was allowed to be given to newborns in hospitals, a huge obstacle to overcome. I was hoping to report his findings in this book, as I believe the outcome will answer many questions, but you'll have to look for the results in *The Lancet* in 2010 (or so Dr. Plummer promised).

Eczema is a first symptom of a potential allergy—and you now understand allergy more from the previous explanation. In my own practice, I tell parents that any rash or eczema indicates that something's going on internally, not just on the surface of the skin. Using cortisone or steroid cream as treatment clears the skin reaction on the surface (suppressing the symptoms) but doesn't deal with why the rash was there in the first place. Often, the rash will disappear for a while (even years) and then reappear in another place on the body. Some children with asthma first had eczema and were treated with cortisone cream, which got rid of the rash but sent the problem to another organ to try to get rid of it—in the case of asthma, the lungs. The inflammation that's first seen on the skin is the body's way of trying to excrete something through one organ, the skin, and when that's unsuccessful, it tries to eliminate it using the lungs and inflammation known as asthma. In my years of consulting, I've seen first-hand this progression in children with asthma. Eczema is multicausal and usually involves several factors, including *candida*, food allergies and sensitivities, poor digestion, too much bad bacteria in the gut, an unhealthy diet, and nutritional deficiencies. I see eczema a lot in my practice, and most often it's the direct result of food allergy or sensitivity, the biggest culprits being wheat, dairy, soy, corn, peanuts, eggs, and sugar. In addition to other recommendations, I often advise removing these allergenic foods and supplementing with probiotics to help support the immune system. It's best to see a nutritionist and/or a naturopath to assess your baby's individual situation and treat the problem. I've seen improvement with using probiotics without diet modifications, but eczema can come back with a cold, flu, or teething.

THE MOST COMMON FOOD ALLERGIES

There are many possible food allergies, but the most common ones are to milk and dairy products, eggs, peanuts, wheat, corn, soy, tree nuts (for example, hazelnuts, walnuts, pecans), beef, sesame, fish, and shellfish. It's the protein within these foods that the immune system reacts to.

The beta-lactoglobulin milk protein, found in whey, is the most common protein that infants and children react to. Casein is also an allergen for some, more so in the case of autism. The father of Pablum (fortified cereal), Dr. Alan Brown, was physician-in-chief at the Hospital for Sick Children in Toronto from 1919 to 1951. He was convinced that feeding babies cow's milk was harmful to babies and stated that "cow's milk is for calves."[70] He was completely right—cows produce milk that's meant for their calves, just as women produce breast milk that's perfectly suited for their infants.

INTRODUCING ALLERGENIC FOODS TOO SOON?

Most practitioners, medical or holistic, in North America, the United Kingdom, and Australia will advise that you avoid giving peanuts to your child until age three. But although this might delay the allergy showing, there doesn't seem to be any evidence that this method is helping to reduce the number of peanut allergies. If anything, peanut allergy is on the rise.

A recent study in Israel looked at Jewish primary school–age children in both Israel and the United Kingdom. Over 8000 children were included in this study, which was carried out by questionnaire. The study found that children in the United Kingdom were 10 times more at risk for peanut allergy than children in Israel. Israeli infants are exposed to peanuts from an average age of eight months, whereas UK infants avoid peanuts until closer to age three.[71] Although the study was inconclusive in its findings, at least in terms of changing current recommendations, it does bring up the question of whether it's better to introduce peanuts at an earlier age than three years. I think, however, that before any potential allergy is introduced, the potential for allergies needs to be taken into account. Are the parents or siblings allergic? Are there risk factors, such as eczema or atopic dermatitis? There seems to be a correlation between eczema and type 1 allergies.

Other studies question why in countries such as China, peanuts are consumed regularly without the greater incidence of peanut allergy seen in North America. One study suggested that it was because peanuts are boiled, perhaps taking away some of the allergenic potential, whereas roasting peanuts may increase the allergic potential.[72]

In the case of cow's milk allergy, a recent study looked at the introduction of cow's milk formula to Caesarean and vaginally born babies who were given supplementary formula directly after birth. In this study, 92.5 percent of babies delivered by C-section were exposed to cow's milk protein in the first few days of life, compared to only 50 percent of those delivered vaginally. The study suggested that the use of hydrolyzed-protein formula may reduce this risk.[73] It would have been interesting to have continued the questioning in this study to see if mom was given antibiotics during labour or took probiotics toward the end of her pregnancy.

Obviously, there are many thoughts, theories, and studies to support conflicting arguments as to whether potentially allergenic foods should be introduced early or not. I still think that with the positive evidence suggesting that probiotics help the immune system to develop properly, what have you got to lose by supplementing with infant probiotics? Not much, as far as I can see—only the possibility of avoiding the life-altering situation of food allergies, supporting the proper development of the immune system, and more.

ALLERGY TESTING

The most common test for allergy is the skin prick or scratch test, where a drop of the potential allergen in solution is put on your skin and a scratch is made through the solution with a needle. If you're allergic, inflammation, redness, and itchiness show up. This test is useful for certain types of allergies, mainly inhalant allergies. It doesn't do well with testing for foods as the IgE antibody is found not in the skin, but in other areas of the body—the intestines, for instance. The scratch test fails to detect 50 percent of food allergies.[74] Allergists use the results, along with the patient's history and family potential for allergies, to decide if there's an allergy or not.

The RAST, or radioallergosorbent, test also measures IgE, but in the blood. This is a good test for airborne allergies, such as seasonal allergies or hay fever.

ELISA testing is a method of testing mainly delayed reactions, but IgE reactions (instant allergic responses) as well as IgE, IgA, and IgM reactions do show up. The ELISA test uses components of the immune system and chemicals in the patient's blood to detect immune responses in the body.

FOOD INTOLERANCE OR SENSITIVITY

What's the difference between a food allergy and sensitivity? The distinction is in the way the immune system reacts. Allergy involves IgE antibody production, while intolerance or sensitivity most commonly involves IgG antibody production. The term *sensitivity* is often used as a catch-all for both allergy and intolerance, but to avoid confusion, I'll use the term *intolerance* for all IgG reactions.

Doctors are not so quick to accept that the IgG reactions millions suffer with are real. Food intolerance doesn't show up with medical testing and therefore isn't often recognized as a problem. Intolerance reactions are not life-threatening, but they can reduce quality of life. Symptoms are generally delayed in showing, unlike with allergies, sometimes taking up to 72 hours to present. By that time you've forgotten what you ate three days ago, making it hard to pinpoint the offending food.

INTOLERANCE SYMPTOMS

Food intolerance is different from allergy not only in having delayed but also in less severe symptoms. Some symptoms of intolerance are similar to those of allergy, making it that much more confusing to diagnose.

Food intolerance symptoms include colic, persistent diarrhea, recurrent ear infections, asthma, stomach aches, rash on the body, bum, or face, dark circles under the eyes, runny nose or what seems a constant cold, eczema, hives, infant insomnia, bedwetting, headache, migraine, fatigue, hyperactivity in children, depression, anxiety, recurrent mouth ulcers or canker sores, aching muscles, vomiting, nausea, and stomach and duodenal ulcers.

As you can see from this list, just about any symptom can be attributed to a food intolerance. Although there are tests for intolerance, the gold standard is to remove a suspected food for at least four weeks and then reintroduce with a large serving. If your symptoms return, there's a good chance you've found the culprit. However, you may have realized already that you felt better for not eating that food during its elimination.

Quite often intolerated foods are those that you crave. The reaction in the body actually gives you a natural high after eating an intolerated food, usually leading you to consume it more.

COMMON FOOD INTOLERANCES

The most common, well-known intolerance is to lactose found in milk. The deficiency of the lactase enzyme leads to the inability to digest lactose, the milk sugar, resulting in a wide variety of symptoms that often differ between individuals. Although lactose is naturally present in breast milk, most of the population stops manufacturing the lactase enzyme between age two (when most babies are weaned) and adolescence. Carolee Bateson-Koch comments, "This is why 70% of the world population is lactase deficient."[75] When you think about it, cow's milk is produced for nursing calves (who weigh about 80 to 100 pounds at birth), not adult humans. I would argue that maybe we aren't meant to drink milk and that it's in fact normal to be lactose intolerant!

Other potentially intolerated foods include wheat, dairy products, soy, corn, nuts, yeast, alcohol, sugar, red meat, eggs, and caffeine. Another complication with food intolerance is that it may take a lot of a particular food before you show symptoms. The most commonly intolerated foods, wheat and dairy, are eaten many times a day, sometimes every day. Our bodies were not meant to eat the same food on a regular basis. I commonly see problems with dairy in infants or toddlers at age one as they move on to milk as a replacement for formula. The slow introduction of cow's milk may not produce a reaction straight away, giving a false sense of security. As the milk intake increases, symptoms start to show, but as nothing showed up when it was first given, it's not suspected as the problem.

Any food can be a problem, especially when you take into consideration the health of the digestive system, the potential for leaky gut from taking antibiotics, or the early introduction of solid food.

WHAT CAN BE DONE ABOUT FOOD ALLERGIES AND INTOLERANCE?

The only way to "cure" an allergy is to re-establish tolerance or prevent loss of tolerance in the first place. Big words for a big problem. See below for some possibilities.

- Be proactive—give probiotics. There is a 50 percent chance that the potential for allergy may be reduced. Remember that the good bacteria colony in the digestive system pushes the developing immune system to respond normally. Give your baby an infant HMF Natogen until about age one and then an adult powder (HMF Powder) until at least age two. Take a potent probiotic while you're pregnant also to ensure there's a strong colony present before baby is born (see chart in Chapter 3, page 57).

- Don't be too clean—put away the sanitizer and antibacterial products. The immune system needs to be challenged with some unsavoury "dirt." Washing hands, floors, and toys is important, but don't go overboard.

- Stay away from sugar—sugar, even in small quantities and especially in small bodies, reduces the strength of the immune system for up to eight hours.

- Avoid giving cow's milk, as it's one of the highest allergenic foods, and avoid giving dairy products until at least one year. If your baby is on formula, investigate hydrolyzed or organic formula (see Chapter 5), and deal with any reactions to a new formula immediately.

- Allow the leaky gut to heal—babies are born with a leaky gut and need time for it to mature. Start solids at six months of age or later if mom or dad has allergies. It's a myth that solid food before six months helps your baby sleep better.

- If eczema appears, figure it out—it may be a sign of greater risk of allergy. So if you see it, adjust your diet if breastfeeding to eliminate common allergenic foods such as dairy, or investigate what the cause might be if your baby's on formula or solid food. Note when it started and whether it correlates with an immunization or medication.

- Avoid antibiotics unless there's no alternative—antibiotics annihilate the good bacteria in the intestines, leaving them exposed to foreign invaders and bad bacteria. Find a good naturopath, homeopath, or nutritionist who can teach you what to do in the case of different types of sickness.

- Eat organic—pesticides and herbicides weaken the immune system and increase the toxicity in your baby. Also, when any plant grows in soil that is fertilized with natural methods, for example, compost in organic farming, naturally occurring beneficial bacteria are present. Pesticides kill off these beneficial bacteria.

- Take immune-boosting vitamins—A, C, E, all the B vitamins including B12 and folic acid, and the minerals zinc and copper allow the army to function at full strength. Take these as part of a multinutrient if breastfeeding, or offer some vitamin C powder mixed with water or food for your baby. Vitamin C shouldn't be given directly to newborns.

POSSIBLE TREATMENTS

For the treatment of allergies, neutralization or desensitization treatment looks promising. Researchers are still conducting trials on small groups of children. Oral immunotherapy (OIT) has successfully treated a small group of children with peanut allergy in the United Kingdom, who were able to tolerate up to 10 peanuts without any adverse consequence. This approach requires medical treatment and should never be tried at home.

I've come across another very accessible treatment that seems to help both allergies and intolerances. The results of the treatment depend on the individual, and success should be discussed with the practitioner. It's known as Bioenergetic Intolerance Elimination, or BIE for short. I got the lowdown from Janet Neilson, a homeopath who uses it in her practice:

> It's essentially electro-acupuncture—no needles—used to clear symptoms of allergies or sensitivities to substances (food, pollens, chemicals, etc.). The device carries energetic frequency information (via a small probe) about various allergens or sensitivities through to the immune system via acupuncture points. These points are like little doorways into the body. The stimulation of these points (for 20 seconds) presents the immune system with information to counter or cancel out its typical response to a food or substance that it's normally sensitive to. For example, cat hair cancels out a cat hair reaction and wheat cancels out a wheat reaction.[76]

Check out www.inht.ca for more information.

8

MAKING HOMEMADE BABY FOOD

Making your own baby food is simple and rewarding. Knowing what goes into your baby's food and feeding nutrient-packed foods with intense flavours is crucial for expanding baby's palate.

Unlike setting up baby's nursery, setting up your kitchen for making baby food is easy. First, make sure that you have knives, utensils, and small appliances that you *love* to work with. Making your own baby and toddler food takes a bit of time, but having the right tools will make the job faster and easier. You won't be motivated to cook a batch of butternut squash if your peeler doesn't work well; likewise, you'll put off chopping carrots if it takes you 20 minutes because your knife is dull. Invest in a few good tools, and you'll be away to the races.

The list below includes everything you need to make baby food. You might have some of these in your kitchen already, but if not, talk to friends to see which products they like, so you don't have to buy three peelers before you find one that works really well.

ESSENTIAL TOOLS FOR MAKING BABY FOOD

- Chopping board
- Chef's knife
- Paring knife (for cutting small fruit and vegetables)
- Peeler

- Stainless steel steamer that sits on top of your saucepan, or bamboo steamer
- Large glass, stainless steel, or "safe" plastic bowl
- Hand blender, food processor, or food mill
- Tasting spoons
- Serving spoon
- Baby food storage trays and containers (I like So Easy Storage Trays)
- Freezer bags for storing food

CHOPPING BOARD

A good-size chopping board, either plastic or wood, is a must. Chopping boards made with food-grade plastic are safe and can be easily cleaned and sanitized. Whichever board you use, make sure there are no deep grooves or cuts in them, as bacteria will make a happy home in there and can transfer to your food. A good rule is to have one chopping board for raw meats and fish and one for only fruits and vegetables. I have a wooden one for fruits, veggies, and bread and a plastic one for raw meat and fish that I put in the dishwasher for a good, hot clean. Wash wooden boards with hot, soapy water, then sanitize when needed with a mixture of 1 tsp (5 mL) bleach (or peroxide, as a "green" option) and 3 cups (750 mL) water. Rinse and air-dry completely after every use.

CHEF'S KNIFE, PARING KNIFE, AND PEELER

A chef's knife is essential for all cooking. You want to make sure it's a sharp knife that feels good in your hand, both in terms of the weight and its handle. If you aren't confident with a big eight-inch (20 cm) chef's knife, there are knives that are less intimidating in size, between six and seven inches (15 to 18 cm). It's worth checking out the knife section of a store such as Ikea to test a few before buying a new one. Contrary to what most people think, more accidents are caused by dull knives than sharp ones as you have to use more pressure and then, *whoops,* the knife slips! A paring knife is for slicing small fruit or cutting out the cores.

When you first make food for your baby, starting around six months, you'll need to peel almost all the fruits and vegetables, as the peel provides too much texture. So, a good peeler is crucial. I searched high and low for an excellent peeler for my Mommy Chef cooking classes, before my mother-in-law gave me a Star brand peeler. The peeler blade is horizontal rather than vertical, and it's the best peeler you'll ever find, so search it out online at www.sproutright.com or at home shows. It's worth the effort.

STAINLESS STEEL STEAMER BASKET OR BAMBOO STEAMER

Choose a bamboo or stainless steel double boiler–type steamer. A double boiler steamer sits high above the bottom of the saucepan, allowing you to put lots of water in the pot, so there's less chance of your saucepan boiling dry. For this reason, I don't suggest the "flower" type baskets that sit inside the saucepan—you can't fit enough water in there to steam carrots for 30 minutes.

The first foods you'll make will be steamed fruits and vegetables. Steaming is preferable over boiling, baking, or microwaving because it helps to retain more nutrients and, if the food's not oversteamed, more water content (especially versus baking). Microwaving is too intense and zaps nutrients, creates hot spots, kills the energy of the produce, and can also change the texture. If you boiled the chopped fruit or vegetable in water, you'd have to drain the liquid and lose the nutrients that leached into the water. If the food is puréed with all the liquid, it would probably end up being too watery. Have you ever heard of boiling a zucchini? Ugh! You get my point.

BOWLS

Once you've steamed your fruits and veggies, you'll put them in a bowl and purée them to get the right texture for your baby. Use a glass, stainless steel, or "safe" (BPA-free) plastic bowl. Glass bowls are preferable—they're a great shape and are really durable (but don't tap the side of one with a hand blender, as it might chip). Plastic might get stained from carrots, beets, and blueberries, and stainless steel bowls can sometimes be too shallow, making it difficult to use your hand blender without the purée ending up all over you and the walls.

HAND BLENDER

A hand or immersion blender is fast and effective and can be used for many foods other than purée. It makes introducing different textures easier, as you can just mash the harder lumps in the purée as you transition to lumps and bumps at around nine months. It's a cinch to clean and easy to travel with, too. I suggest saving your normal blender for making smoothies, since puréeing food in a blender requires water, and unless you know exactly how much to add, you have to continually stop the machine to push down food from the top to the bottom. Too time-consuming! A food mill is great for making small batches of purée, but it would take a while to do a steamer basket full of sweet potato, for instance. Some purées can also be made in a food processor, but larger amounts of liquid tend to spill out of the bowl, leaving you with more mess to clean up.

BABY FOOD STORAGE TRAYS AND CONTAINERS

So Easy Storage Trays are my favourite—they're durable and contain no bisphenol A, PVC, or phthalates. They're similar to ice cube trays but have lids and are made of high-quality plastic without harmful toxins. If you're using an ice cube tray for freezing, check the quality of the plastic first.

Once your food is frozen, run the back of the tray under hot water (they don't bend or twist like other trays because of the type of plastic used) and dump the cubes into a freezer bag for storage. This way you have the trays empty for your next batch of food and only need to purchase two to four trays.

Some people like to store their baby food in the individual containers (usually 2 oz cups) because they can just move them from the freezer to the refrigerator to defrost or take them along when they're on the go. To keep your food in this type of container, you'll need to have more on hand or pop out each one as it freezes rather than one full tray at a time. This can be more time-consuming, and they can leak. A good idea, but maybe not worth the extra trouble.

FREEZER BAGS FOR STORING FOOD

Once you've frozen your baby food into either trays or individual containers, pop it out and store each batch in a freezer bag, making sure to label and date the bag.

Try to get as much air out as possible to reduce freezer burn. The food can be kept in a fridge freezer for up to three months, or longer in a chest freezer, as the door isn't opened as often. Most freezer bags are made from polyethylene so should be fine for use with cold foods like frozen baby food cubes.

SHOPPING FOR FRUITS AND VEGETABLES

Fruits and vegetables are the first foods your baby will eat and, ideally, will continue to eat as he gets older. Shopping for what's best has become confusing with the movements toward buying local and organic. Which do you choose? If possible, I would try to get local, seasonal, and organic produce. When you buy locally, not only are you supporting your local farmers and economy, but also a shorter travel time means food that is fresher, more nutritious, tastier, and better for the environment. Often the foods sold at your local farmers' market were picked within 24 hours of purchase.

Buying what's local and in season means that you're eating foods when they're at their peak for taste and nutrients and when they're in abundance, so they cost less than when out of season.

ORGANIC

Try to buy organic as much as possible. Any amount of organic food given to your baby or toddler is better than none. See page 149 for a list of the most important foods to buy organic and those that are not sprayed as much so are safer to buy conventional.

The taste of organic fruit and vegetables is often more intense—in other words, more delicious. The only downside to organic is that fresh produce doesn't always keep as long and is often bruised and irregularly shaped so not as visually appealing. But it's fun for children to see unusual shapes. We've seen carrots that look like hands with five fingers. It all creates more interest in food, which is never a bad thing.

Organic foods are naturally grown without the use of synthetically manufactured chemical fertilizers, pesticides, herbicides, fungicides, antibiotics, and hormones or genetically modified organisms (GMs). A staggering five to six billion pounds of insecticides, herbicides, fungicides, rodenticides, and other synthetic chemicals are applied throughout the world every year.[77] The Pesticide Action Network website explains the health concerns associated with conventional foods: "chronic health effects can result from low dose exposure to pesticides over time. Even extremely low doses of pesticides, particularly during foetal development, infancy and childhood, are linked to cancers, birth defects, developmental delays, asthma, and Parkinson's disease."[78]

Introducing organic foods as your baby's first foods is especially important because the immaturity of your baby's developing systems leaves her vulnerable to chemicals, which eventually may overload it. This could increase the likelihood of intolerances and adverse reactions in susceptible babies.

Organic farming is also better for the environment as it uses compost and other natural fertilizers that make the soil rich with life, and organic farming helps keep the ecosystem healthy and alive.

CONVENTIONAL

Conventional food is what you'll find at most supermarkets (that is, anything that's not labelled organic). It's produced using a variety of pest management techniques, including crop rotation, tillage, pesticides, and crop nutrients such as manure and synthetic fertilizers. Research shows that conventional food may not be as healthy because of the chemicals used, as well as the lower nutrient content. Refer to page 149 for a list of safer conventional foods.

FROZEN

Frozen fruits and vegetables are convenient and are a great way to have out-of-season foods on hand without spoilage. Produce that you find frozen has been picked and then flash-frozen to maintain its nutrients. If you grow fruits and vegetables in your garden, freeze them for future use. It may be worth packaging your harvest with a vacuum sealer to eliminate the chances of freezer burn.

CANNED

Use canned fruits and vegetables as a last resort. They're often high in sugar and salt and extremely low in enzymes and nutrients. Some cans are lined with bisphenol A, which can leach into your food—this is especially true of canned tomatoes. Canned beans (such as Eden Organics beans) usually have an enamel lining so are safe to use and very handy.

CLEANING FRUITS AND VEGETABLES

Although you'll need to peel most fruits and vegetables for your baby or toddler, they still need to be washed before consuming or cooking. Bacteria can cross from the peeler or knife into the food. In addition, washing can help reduce the amount of pesticides, soil lead, and pathogens on produce.

WASHING TIPS

- Wash produce under clean, running water. Don't skip this step!
- Use a vegetable scrub brush or pad on produce with a firm skin, such as carrots, potatoes, melons, and squash.
- Discard outer leaves of leafy greens or dense vegetables such as broccoli, cauliflower, and brussels sprouts. Soak in water for a few minutes to dislodge dirt, and rinse thoroughly under running water.
- Soak herbs such as parsley and cilantro for 15 minutes, then rinse thoroughly.
- Soap and chlorine wash can leave residues, so it's better to avoid them. Special produce washes remove chemical residues, but they don't kill bacteria or mould. Wash hands with soap to avoid cross-contamination from preparing other foods or after wiping your nose or visiting the bathroom.

STORING FRUITS AND VEGETABLES

- Fruits and vegetables are best consumed fresh, so try to buy them every two to three days if possible. If produce sits in your fridge for two weeks it loses a lot of nutrients as well as flavour.
- Refrigerate leafy vegetables wrapped in a tea towel and washed fruits and vegetables in cloth bags, which helps lengthen their shelf life.
- Mushrooms are best stored in paper bags so that they can breathe.
- Store onions, garlic, and potatoes in a cool, dark, dry place.

- When you get home from shopping, wash all your fruits so they're ready to eat. Put them in a bowl on the counter where they won't be forgotten!

NOW YOU'VE GOT THE GEAR—START COOKING!

Making your own baby food is fast, easy, and economical. For some reason, there's a misconception that homemade baby food is a lot of work, but it's really so easy and worth the time for all the great benefits it gives your baby.

Preparing your own food allows you to choose exactly what goes into it and to customize it to suit the tastes of your baby. You decide on the food combinations to create new tastes and flavours, and you can adjust the food to give it chunkier textures as your baby gets older.

The taste and texture from food made at home exposes your baby to *real food* that will eventually be served at family meals. Making your own food may also prevent picky eating, as you know your child's likes and dislikes and can work to expand his palate. And when was the last time you saw cilantro, parsley, garlic, or ginger in a jar? Remember that it can take 8 to 12 times before your baby takes to a particular flavour or food. So keep trying it!

Cooking for Age 6 to 9 Months

I recommend butternut squash and pear as baby's first foods—they are the perfect taste and texture for new palates. After that you can follow the list in no particular order, alternating with different coloured vegetables and fruits. Mix it up!

Vegetables	Fruits
Asparagus	Apples
Beets	Apricots
Broccoli	Avocado
Butternut squash	Banana
Carrots	Blueberries
Cauliflower	Cherries
Green beans	Dried apricots
Green peas	Mango
Parsnips	Papaya
Sweet potato	Pears
Turnip	Plums
Zucchini	Prunes (dried plums)

How to Prepare First Foods

1. Peel, core, and chop the fruit or vegetable into small cubes. The smaller you chop them, the faster they'll cook. Adjust the steaming time depending on the size.

2. Fill up your saucepan with enough water so that it won't boil away, keeping in mind that harder vegetables such as carrots and beets take longer to steam. Put the pot on the stove on high and bring to a boil with the lid on to heat it up faster.

3. Put your chopped food into the steamer basket and place on top of the boiling water. Turn down the heat from high to medium so the water doesn't boil over.

4. Steam with the lid on until fruits or vegetables are tender. You'll know they're cooked when a knife can slide through the food or they can be easily mashed without any resistance.

5. Empty the contents into a bowl suitable for puréeing.

6. Purée by mashing with your hand (immersion) blender or food processor *before* adding any water.

7. Add water, a scant 1/4 cup (50 mL) at a time. As you make more food for your baby you'll learn roughly how much water you need, but for now add it in slowly (see the recipes at the end of Chapter 9 for approximate amounts).

8. Keep puréeing until it's the texture of a smooth, thick soup for first meals. As your baby gets older, add a bit less water to your purée and leave a few lumps or bumps in it.

Some vegetables are more fibrous than others, including sweet potato and parsnips, and will need more water. Add 1/4 to 1/2 cup (50 mL to 125 mL) water, and expect to add about 1 to 2 cups (250 mL to 500 mL) for a large batch. Every fruit and vegetable will need different amounts of water, so be sure to mash it first to see the consistency if you haven't made it before. The added water not only creates a texture that your baby can swallow, but with some of the more fibrous vegetables, helps move the fibre through baby's digestive system easily, lessening the chance of constipation.

Note: Dried fruit such as apricots or prunes should be boiled with enough water to cover them in the saucepan, until they become plump. Add the water in the saucepan to the purée, using extra if you're freezing it.

Mash and Serve

Ripe banana, avocado, and papaya can be mashed with a fork or the back of a spoon and served. They're great foods for on the go. As your baby gets older and more accustomed to texture, you can purée pear and blueberry without steaming.

To Peel or Not to Peel

- Peel the first foods for your baby—the skin gives more texture that might not be well received. As she gets older, you can try leaving the skin on pear, apple, and sweet potato, being sure to wash it well.
- Always peel the skin of butternut squash, sweet potato, apple, and pear.
- Scrub or peel carrots, beets, parsnips, and turnips.
- Peel the stalk of broccoli and chop it to yield more.
- Don't peel zucchini, plums, apricots, nectarines, blueberries, and green beans or take the skin off peas.
- Chop cauliflower and remove the stalk.
- Take the peel off avocado, banana, mango, and papaya.

- Any of the above can be used frozen, if applicable. Frozen wild blueberries, for example, are available all year and are usually cheaper than fresh.

A Word about Water

Each batch of food may need more or less water to get the right consistency. Always mash the food before adding water to avoid making it too runny. As you become an expert at making purée, you'll become more confident about adding water without measuring.

Add the most water: more than 1 cup (250 mL) for half a steamer basket or more	Add a medium amount of water: ½ to 1 cup (125 to 250 mL) for half a steamer basket or more	Add a bit of water: ½ cup (125 mL) or less	No water needed
Beets, parsnips, sweet potato	Broccoli, butternut squash, carrots, cauliflower, dried apricots, green beans	Apples, blueberries, fresh apricots, mango, nectarines	Avocado, banana, papaya, pear, plum, zucchini

We usually take lot of care when choosing the types and quality of food for our babies, but we often don't give water as high a priority. I highly recommend using filtered water to drink or add to baby's food. Depending on the filter, it can remove contaminants of bacteria, spores, lead, chlorine, and other pollutants, including medication. Filters range from Brita to reverse osmosis water filtration systems. Check out the resource section for websites to research further and find a water filter that suits your budget and needs.

See the end of Chapter 9 for recipes for six- to nine-month-olds.

From the Mouths of Moms

I had problems breastfeeding, so for me making baby food for my son was something that was easy and empowering. It's a good excuse to buy a fancy food processor. Plus, you can impress other people with your mother goddess skills—they don't have to know how easy it is!

—KATIE, MOM OF ONE

PREPARING NEXT-STAGE FOODS (9 TO 12 MONTHS)

At this stage, the method of cooking changes from steaming most purées to cooking in a saucepan to make more of a stew-like meal. All foods can still be puréed to the texture your baby likes, and little by little you can purée a bit less, leaving a few lumps or bumps, or reducing the amount of water to create a thicker purée.

This is the stage at which I see most parents start down a road that they didn't necessarily want to go down, as finger foods become a more important part of baby's diet. If you've been using jarred food, you might find that you need to wean your baby on to the flavourful recipes in Chapter 10. Start with a bit of what he knows and likes, adding in a teaspoon at a time of the new food to give him time to get used to it.

My general guideline is to introduce textured purées around nine months of age, although your baby might be ready for lumpier food earlier. Try introducing it to your baby, but if she "gags" she's not ready; simply try it again in a couple of weeks.

At this stage you're going to slowly increase the texture of baby's food each week or so. This is where the wonderful versatility of making your own baby food comes into play. Start slowly and give your baby time to get used to the new texture in his mouth.

The purées you make for this age will include a wider variety of fruits and vegetables, all cooked in the same saucepan. You'll also start giving legumes (beans, peas, and lentils), brown rice, and gluten-free grains and seeds, which are high in fibre, protein, iron, and many other vitamins and minerals. Baby's digestive system has matured a lot since the first introduction of food at six months, so he's ready at this stage to eat these foods.

To make the purées, peel, core, and chop fruit or vegetables into small cubes. Add these to a saucepan with water or organic stock (no sodium) and a choice of legumes (beans, peas, and lentils), brown rice, and gluten-free grains and seeds. Simmer until the fruits or vegetables are tender and the grain, bean, or legume is well cooked.

Empty into a bowl suitable for puréeing, and mash with your hand blender. If the mixture is too thick, add water to thin it out. Remember that you can always add more water (or even breast milk or formula) upon serving if it's too thick. As your baby gets older, you can adjust the texture by "pulsing" the hand blender to create a little more texture with lumps and bumps. And when she's close to toddler age, you might not even have to purée her food.

The list below outlines the order to follow in making the recipes in Chapter 10, as they go from least texture to most texture. At any time you can give your baby steamed vegetable finger foods in the order suggested below. See Chapter 10 for a full list of finger foods (other than fruits and vegetables) as well as dips.

TEXTURED PURÉES

The Next Stage: 9- to 12-month-olds transitioning to chunkier meals	Super-Chunky: 10 months and older or when baby is ready for full texture without puréeing
Introduction to Lentils	Baby's First Chicken or Turkey
Cheeky Chickpeas	Delicious Lentil Dahl
Sweet Potato Purée	Bean and Rice Surprise
Immune Boosting Purée	Brown Rice Pudding
Amazing Sweet Amaranth	Fruity Curry Buckwheat
Introducing ... Quinoa	

FINGER FOODS

Steamed Finger Foods	Other Finger Foods
Cauliflower	Finger Food Pancakes
Broccoli	Hummus
Green Beans	Beany Green Dip
Carrots	Yummy Carrot Spread
Asparagus	
Beets	

Storage

To store baby's food, let it cool and then spoon it into bisphenol-A–free baby food trays or cubes and freeze for at least 24 hours. Once frozen, pop out the frozen food into a storage freezer bag, and label it with the contents and date on the outside of the bag. Prepared food will keep in the refrigerator for three days, and in the freezer for up to three months.

Foods to Buy Organic

Although I highly recommend feeding babies exclusively organic foods to limit their toxic load, I understand that not everyone will be able to fit this into their

budget. The Environmental Working Group, a nonprofit organization, has ana-
lyzed the results of nearly 87,000 tests for pesticides on produce collected by the
U.S. Department of Agriculture and the U.S. Food and Drug Administration
between 2000 and 2007. The result is a list that ranks the most commonly contaminated produce and the least contaminated. Use this list to help decide which
fruits and vegetables to buy or not buy organic.

SHOPPER'S GUIDE TO PESTICIDES

Dirty Dozen Buy These Organic	Clean 15 Lowest in Pesticides
Peach	Onion
Apple	Avocado
Bell pepper	Sweet corn (remember that nonorganic is GM)
Celery	Pineapple
Nectarine	Mango
Strawberries	Asparagus
Cherries	Sweet peas
Kale	Kiwi
Lettuce	Cabbage
Grapes (imported)	Eggplant
Carrot	Papaya
Pear	Watermelon
	Broccoli
	Tomato
	Sweet potato

Source: Environmental Working Group, 2009, "Shopper's Guide to Pesticides," www.foodnews.org.

FIRST FOODS
A Healthy Start with 6- to 9-Month Purée Recipes

Starting your baby on solids can be a daunting and yet exciting time. There's a lot of conflicting advice available, not to mention the opinion of others: mom, mother-in-law, friends, the internet, and, of course, your doctor. Here, I'll break down weaning on to solid food into easy steps and explain why you'll introduce certain foods at different times. And don't forget, you're not alone—you'll read about other new moms' experiences too.

WHEN TO START SOLIDS

Both Health Canada and the World Health Organization recommend exclusively breastfeeding for the first six months of your baby's life. Breast milk provides all the nutrition your baby needs and will continue to do so as solid food is introduced and slowly increased. It's best if you can continue breastfeeding along with solid food until at least one year of age, and morning and evening to age two. The longer you breastfeed, the more your baby will gain the benefits of your own immune antibodies and super-absorbable vitamins, minerals, and enzymes that help her digest the essential fats in breast milk. Breast milk becomes more concentrated in some minerals and proteins as your baby starts to breastfeed less when solids increase to ensure that she's still getting everything she needs.[79] Bottle-fed babies should also be fed formula exclusively, without solid food, until six months, and this will remain the main source of nutrition until age one.

Before you set up the high chair and choose the bib and bowl with matching spoon, sit down and read this, absorb it, and let it be your new mantra during this new chapter in your lives: introducing solids is all about the *introduction of solids*. Baby, meet spoon with new taste, texture, and colour on it. This is a whole new experience for your baby, so don't expect that it will all go according to

Reaction Confusion

Be sure to start food on a day when your baby is healthy, with no colds or viruses, teething episodes, or recent vaccinations. These can complicate the smooth introduction to solids, as your baby may suffer symptoms including rash, fever, or out-of-sorts behaviour.

plan (you might have learned that once or twice in the past six months). The whole process is new, from the food coming toward him on a spoon, rather from the breast or bottle, to the new taste and thicker texture, the need for his digestive system to work on something other than "milk" (breast or formula), and then having to poo it out. It's new inside and out. And the amount of food your baby eats to begin with could be literally a thimbleful. You're not alone if you think it's hardly worth the time and effort to purée carrots, but remember, she'll eat it eventually, if not on the first or second try, maybe the fifth. If you've come across a strict schedule of when introducing solids should happen, with time of day and

how much she should be eating, throw it out. It's too much pressure for your baby to live up to those expectations, and feeding often doesn't go to schedule. Even if my recommendation of when to start and progress with solids isn't going well, change it until you see success.

Your baby may show signs that he's ready to start on solids at four or five months (see below); however, it's best to wait until he's six months old because the digestive system is continuing to mature. This maturity may reduce the risk of allergies. Every baby

Adding Cereal to the Bottle: A Bad Idea

Myth: Mixing rice cereal in your baby's bottle before he's four months old will help him sleep. Fact: If you offer any food other than breast milk or formula before four months of age, you run the risk of increasing the potential for allergies, digestive complaints, and skin rashes and slowing down the maturation of the digestive tract. Don't do it—that tiny digestive system isn't ready yet.

is different in his eagerness to start, so assess your own situation, but don't be fooled into starting too early.

"I Want Food" Signs

- Baby shows interest in your plate, tries to grab your food or cutlery, or has a new interest in what's happening at the table.
- She mimics your eating or mouth motions.
- She can sit up on her own.
- The tongue's sucking reflex has relaxed. Food will be able to pass into the throat.
- Your baby seems less satisfied with breastfeeding or formula, which means she may need more calories (from food). This doesn't indicate that you're not producing enough breast milk or not offering enough formula.

If your baby shows these signs between four and six months and you're tempted to start with solids earlier than six months, give it time (and don't forget that cereals are also considered solids—see "The Cereal Debate" later in the chapter). Your baby won't starve by sticking with breast milk or formula. Keep in mind that the digestive system is still maturing and healing its leaky gut, and it needs until six months to do this.

Please don't think that if your baby starts to wake up in the middle of the night it's because he's hungry. Most of the time, that's not the case. It could be that he's uncomfortable from teething or simply has made a slight change in his sleep pattern. However, if you assume that hunger is the reason and begin to nurse or bottle-feed more often in the night, *bang*, you've started a new habit of waking up to feed every two to three hours again. And that's the reason why you're a zombie.

Introducing solids may actually make the sleep situation worse because the digestive system isn't ready—gassiness, constipation, or colic-like symptoms of wailing for hours might result. In a recent online poll of moms, I found that 24 percent of moms tried giving their baby solids to help improve sleeping patterns, but 60 percent said it didn't work, and 7 percent said it made sleep worse.[80]

All too often I see new moms starting solids out of desperation, in the hopes that it will help baby sleep. If it actually worked, there would be a lot of very well-rested new moms, full of energy and without a mention of how much they dread nighttime. In my years of listening to the conversations of new moms, I've found that sleepless nights are the norm. We're all exhausted most of the time and pray for the miracle of a good night's sleep. Tracey Ruiz, also known as "The Sleep Doula," says,

> *One of the most common suggestions my clients are given by medical professionals is "Just wait till they start solids—they'll start sleeping through the night." But to their surprise, after solids are introduced, there is still no change or improvement. A baby or toddler isn't going to eat well during the day if they know they can eat or nurse all night long. I liken it to an all-night buffet, and why would they give up the service? For sleep? Probably not. At around four months they get a new awareness of what's around them, become distracted, maybe nibble during the day as opposed to a full feeding. At night you see them starting waking every two to three hours. What is given to put them to sleep— breast, bottle or something else—they will need that same tool to go back to sleep again in the middle of the night. A very high percentage of sleep problems are due to habit, not hunger.[81]*

TIME OF DAY TO START

Although the success of solids is not always to do with your baby's hunger, for breastfed babies, starting later in the day may be better. For some moms, but not all, breast milk stores are lower later in the afternoon, so offering solids around this time is what I advise. Breakfast seems to be the least successful meal to start with; in fact, it might be the last meal of the three that you introduce. Formula-fed babies can start at either lunch or dinner as their milk intake is usually more scheduled than on demand.

Caution with Potentially Allergenic Foods

When introducing potentially allergenic foods—egg yolk, nuts and seeds, dairy products, and strawberries—between nine months and one year, be sure to allow at least five hours between the time you give the food and bedtime so you can be sure there's no adverse reaction. If there are allergies in the family, delay the start of most of the above foods until after one year.

Start with either an 11 a.m. to 12 noon lunch or 4 to 5 p.m. dinner, depending on when your baby goes to bed for the night. Pick one of these times, and if it isn't working, try another time of day.

MILK FIRST, THEN FOOD

Because your baby's breast milk or formula ("milk") is her main source of nutrition, I recommend continuing with your routine milk feed and offering food after. The solids are extra calories and nutrients *on top of* her usual daily nutrient intake from milk. Remember that this is about trying out food as opposed to getting nutrients from it, and you don't want to take away from the nutrition that comes from milk. So nurse or bottle-feed your baby as usual, be sure she has had a nap and isn't tired, and within an hour of the milk feeding, give her a meal of solids. That hour is just a guideline to give you enough time to change a diaper, get the food ready, warm it if you need to, get baby comfortable, and sit down to feed her. Change the timing between nursing and food depending on your baby and her schedule. And if your baby isn't interested in her solids after milk, it may not be because she's already full. Some babies are slow to start when introducing food.

As his food intake increases, you may notice that your baby starts to nurse less or leave an ounce or two in his bottle. This is his way of weaning himself off milk as his food intake increases. Let him be in charge of this unless he refuses milk because of a fast introduction of solids. Moving too quickly away from milk might leave him deficient in certain nutrients, as it provides him with protein, fat, carbohydrates, vitamins, minerals, and antibodies (in breast milk). You won't find all that in two tablespoons of butternut squash!

HOW MUCH TO START WITH

Remember, this is more about the experience than about nourishment. Your baby may start with a fingertip of food to a tablespoon of food—really, that's all you can expect at the beginning. Whatever she chooses to take, start slowly. If your baby takes to this like a duck to water, then you have to be in charge of the amount, or you might see what you've just served come right back up. That small stomach will only hold so much, so if after two tablespoons your baby is still keen, I might suggest slowing down the pace. If one teaspoon is taken in and swallowed, you're off to a great start. You might not have seen rejection, but perhaps a funny face or two.

A few years ago, I held one of my regular workshops at Whole Foods Market in Toronto about introducing your baby to solids. I always start by having the moms or dads introduce themselves and their babies—name, baby's name, age, breastfed or formula-fed, and whether they've started solids yet. One of the attendees introduced herself and her baby and proudly shared with the group that her baby had started solids the day before. She started with rice cereal, and baby loved it so much that mom offered the cereal three times that day. She was relieved that it went well and excited to keep going. I suggested that she start slowly to allow her baby's digestive system to get accustomed to digesting solids. But I could tell that she wasn't convinced, as things had gone so well. About 15 minutes later, her baby started crying. And she cried inconsolably for the rest of the hour-long workshop. Mom was obviously concerned and at a loss as to what was going on. She told the group that her baby was never like this. I watched her efforts to calm her, and it really didn't matter what mom did—put her down, pick her up, rock her, bounce her, nothing was helping. Toward the end of the class, I suggested that perhaps the previous day's rice cereal consumption was not agreeing with her and she was either experiencing a food reaction or it was too much not just for one day, but for the first day of starting solids. Mom agreed and said she would slow the pace down.

The message? Although it's exciting to start solids, you have to go with the pace at which your baby's digestive system can keep up. Slow and steady is really the best way forward for everyone—both for your baby's health and your sanity.

Expect some of the food to end up on your baby's face or hands, and remember it's about the experience, not how much food he actually swallows. If you consistently see his tongue pushing the food out of his mouth, the tongue thrust reflex may not have relaxed, so try again in another week or so. If there are concerns over your baby's lack of weight gain (see "Tipping the Scale," page 161), still take your time—although you want more food

> ### Survey Says ... Success of Solids
>
> In my online survey, 44 percent of moms said that their babies took to solids like a duck to water, 37 percent did well, 12 percent were lukewarm, and 9 percent were not interested.[82]

to go in for a higher calorie intake, your baby may not be able to keep up with as much as you want him to.

To progress, increase the amount of food until you see that your baby's taking a consistent amount, whatever that may be—two to four tablespoons or so. Then you can add another meal—if you started with lunch, add dinner. If dinner was the first meal, give lunch. Breakfast is usually the last meal to add. It may take a number of weeks before you offer a second and then third meal. For instance, offer one meal for two to three weeks, and if that's going well, introduce the next meal. The third meal may not start until well into the second month of solids, around eight or even nine months. I like the "rule" of having your baby on three meals a day by the time she's nine months.

Some babies do well with one meal and the second meal also goes down easily; others can take it or leave it. If another meal isn't going well, leave it for a week or two and try again. There is no set amount that your baby should be eating; although you might come across some recommendations, I usually suggest following your baby's cues. Keep up the same milk intake until she starts to want less. Your baby will let you know.

The amount of food your baby eats on any given day can change dramatically. During a growth spurt, expect the intake to increase; later, it might go back to what it was previously. If a cold or any sickness is coming on or you detect a teething episode, expect a decrease in appetite. You can't force-feed your baby, so try not to worry. Whatever the reason, it usually passes, and although it can take some time to get back to where you once were, you will get there.

STARTING SOLIDS WITH A PLAN

Whichever food you start with—butternut squash, banana, or pear—offer the same food for four or five consecutive days before moving on to a new one. You'll have heard it's recommended to wait three days before trying a new food, but I prefer four to five days. If your baby does have a reaction (and there's no reason to suspect she necessarily will), it's easier to figure out what caused it. Say you start on a Monday with banana, giving it each day until Wednesday. On Thursday morning you start on apple and a rash appears. It could be the apple that was just eaten or the banana from yesterday. Feeding one food for at least four days gives your baby's system time to show a reaction or not. Use the Baby Feeding

Calendar at the end of the chapter to make note of what your baby is drinking and eating and any symptoms.

What Is a Reaction?

For a clear outline of symptoms of allergic reaction and food intolerance or sensitivity, read Chapter 7. But for quick reference, you're looking for anything new or different in your baby. Common symptoms of food sensitivity include a rash on the bum, face, torso, arms—well, just about anywhere—a change in bowel habits (diarrhea or constipation), gassiness, and throwing up or spitting up, but your baby could show different symptoms.

Generally, food allergies show up faster than food intolerance. Allergic reactions take minutes to hours to show and might look like hives, mainly on the trunk of the body, on the face, or both. On the first introduction of an allergenic food, a lesser reaction may take place, but subsequent exposure could lead to stronger reactions. For instance, the first time I gave my daughter egg yolk, at nine months, she broke out in hives all over her body. A month later I tried again, and she violently threw up. I knew it was a problem for her and kept it out of her diet until she was over one year old, and found that because she was older, she could tolerate it. Some allergies can weaken with age, but be sure to check with your doctor before offering any food that has shown a reaction in the past.

Skin reactions such as eczema can appear for the first time, or existing patches may flare up. A bum rash can appear or worsen with the introduction of a sugary food. So be sure to read the label of the food you're about to introduce if you haven't made it yourself.

Food intolerance or sensitivity can take longer to show up, sometimes up to 72 hours, which is why feeding solids may involve some detective work. And if you re-read the reaction symptoms above, they're very similar to symptoms of teething. So it gets tough to keep things straight. When I speak with parents about food reactions, we look back to the days leading up to the symptoms—the answer is usually there somewhere. For example, if your baby has constipation, look back at what she ate over the last three days. Was there an increased amount of a cereal? Did you just start on formula or mix cereal with formula? Either situation could be the cause. The Baby Feeding Calendar at the end of this chapter can help you keep track of the foods you've introduced and any new reactions.

Relying on memory at this point may not be your best strategy (as we saw in Chapter 2, mommy brain is real!).

If you do suspect a reaction to a food, remove it, make a note with a red flag, and leave at least three weeks before trying it again. When you give that food again, make sure there's nothing else going on—recent vaccination, teething, cold, or other sickness. Look for the same symptoms. If they come back, wait three months before reintroducing. Discuss your findings with your doctor for her records and advice (although doctors don't always recognize food intolerance reactions).

THE CEREAL DEBATE

There are different recommendations about which food to start with first; medical doctors say start with baby rice, and more recently meat, but I suggest fruits and vegetables as the food of choice. Let me explain.

Infant cereals are often recommended because they're fortified with iron. Doctors are under the impression that iron stores run out at six months of age, but that may not be the case. A medical student once told me that they're taught in medical school that breast milk contains no iron, so potential iron deficiency in baby's diet is a concern. Yet it's been proven over and over again that the iron in breast milk is in *the* most absorbable form. Breast milk also contains proteins called lactoferrin and transferrin that grab on to the iron so it can be absorbed by baby. Bad bacteria commonly live in the digestive tract and can feed on iron from the diet, leaving baby deficient. This might be more common in formula-fed babies without the supplementation of probiotics (see Chapters 3 and 6). So those iron-fortified cereals (with no lactoferrin or transferrin) may not do what the doctors want them to, especially with common situations of high bad bacteria levels and low beneficial bacteria (particularly after antibiotic use). Iron fortification or supplementation is also linked with constipation—a reaction I often see after cereal is introduced.

After researching which food to start my first daughter on, I found fruits and vegetables the best. I was hesitant about beginning with the usual cereal, having known other babies who were constipated after starting solids, so I was cautious and wanted an alternative for her. Since then, introducing fruits and vegetables first has become more common, and those babies I know who've followed this order are growing up healthy and without iron-deficiency anemia.

The grains in most infant cereals, including rice, oats, and barley, contain starch, which needs to be broken down with enzymes. When babies are born, they haven't yet developed their full spectrum of enzymes, including the carbohydrate (starch) digesting enzymes ptyalin and amylase. Ptyalin, found in saliva in the mouth (also known as salivary amylase), and amylase are specifically needed to digest starches found in cereals. Around six months of age, amylase slowly increases to digest carbohydrate or starchy foods, but not enough is produced to handle the cereals yet.

Giving cereals closer to one year of age is preferable but from a practical standpoint can be difficult to follow through on. The other reason to delay boxed cereal is that it's a processed food and far from its original state. For instance, rice processing removes the bran and outer shell, where most of the nutrients are. During the processing of infant cereal some key nutrients are lost, including iron, and so these products are fortified with iron in the form of ferrum sulfate.

Ferrum sulfate is a fairly absorbable form of iron; however, it's known for its digestive aggravation leading to constipation. I've seen

Cereal: An Old-School Recommendation

Fortified cereal was first recommended in 1931 with the invention of Pablum by Dr. Alan Brown, along with Dr. Fred Tisdall and Dr. Theo Drake, at the Hospital for Sick Children in Toronto. These doctors developed Pablum as a way to reduce the infant death rate by improving nutrition because formula was lacking in the nutrients babies needed to thrive. Their first ready-to-eat cereal was enriched with vitamins A, B1 and B2, D, and E and produced from a mixture of wheat, oats, corn, and bone meal plus wheat germ, dried brewer's yeast, and alfalfa. Although it didn't provide everything that an infant needed, it was a huge hit, and it reduced infant deaths. Pablum, or a version of it, anyway, is still recommended today. Years of research have improved formula—today, it's a high-tech product with more absorbable nutrients.

Survey Says ... First Food

My online survey asked, "What was the first food you started your baby on?" The results showed that 70 percent started on cereal, 55 percent started on vegetables and fruits, and 2 percent started on meat. (Some selected more than one option.)[83]

countless babies unnecessarily suffer with constipation on the introduction of cereal. The pressure to feed cereals and over time, in increasing amounts, leads to chronic constipation in babies who are not yet one year old. Prune or other juices are commonly recommended to ease this common complaint, and if that doesn't help, mineral oil ingestion is the next step (poor babes—that's enough to make anyone feel ill). Why the first suggestion isn't to stop the cereal until the problem rights itself is beyond me. It's the cause of the constipation, so just take it out of the diet and leave it out until your baby is pooing daily.

FIRST FOODS: FRUITS AND VEGGIES

I suggest starting with banana, apple, pear, avocado, carrots, yams or sweet potato, butternut squash, or parsnips. My favourites to start with are butternut squash as the first vegetable and pear as the fruit. It's a common misconception that starting with fruits will predispose your baby to a sweet tooth. But if you want to be on the safe side, start with butternut squash, a sweeter vegetable than broccoli, for instance. In case you haven't tasted breast or formula milk, it's much sweeter than most fruits and vegetables, so starting with a not-so-sweet vegetable such as broccoli may not be the success you hope it to be.

THE NEW FAD: MEAT

Your public health nurse or doctor may recommend meat as the first food. I understand the idea behind this, but sorry, folks, once again I disagree. Meat is a good source of heme iron (with about 40 percent heme iron and the rest non-heme), a more absorbable form of iron from food that's good for your baby, but the benefit stops there. Let me explain.

The good bacteria or *acidophilus* cultures that live in your baby's digestive system become unbalanced with the introduction of meat. The ratio of good to not-so-good bacteria in babies eating fruits and vegetables is 50:50. When meat is introduced it changes to closer to 90 percent unfavourable bacteria and 10 percent good guys. As you may remember from previous chapters, the benefits of good bacteria for your baby include keeping his immune system strong, helping to digest food, synthesizing B vitamins and vitamin K, and helping reduce the incidence of allergies. This is not a balance to upset at such a young age.

High levels of protein in anyone's diet lead to greater acidity, and the body calls on calcium to maintain its alkalinity. When your baby's body is building bone strength by depositing calcium into bones, this isn't the time to increase animal protein for the sake of iron intake.

Dr. George A. Wootan, a family practitioner, medical associate of La Leche League International, and member of the Institute for Functional Medicine, states that "hydrochloric acid—used to digest most protein—doesn't even appear in the stomach until the end of the seventh month and doesn't reach a peak until the eighteenth month."[84] There's a huge drain on digestive energy as the body tries to break down complete proteins it's not ready to cope with.

It's also difficult to purée meat so that it's swallowable and tasty without adding fruits and vegetables. So, the vegetables must come first. At nine months, egg yolk, an iron-rich food, may be offered. If after reading the above you choose to follow your doctor's guidelines regarding giving meat to your baby, wait until she's is at least 10 months old, or, even better, wait until age one.

Foods to Avoid Completely

There are a few foods that are no-nos until age one:

- Egg white is more allergenic than egg yolk.
- Honey may be contaminated with botulism, which your baby's digestive system can't fight off.
- Strawberries may cause an allergic reaction. Kiwi is also allergenic, although less so.
- Tomatoes can be acidic, causing rash on the face or bum.
- Citrus fruits, including oranges and grapefruit, in particular, as they're usually eaten in larger quantity, and limes and lemons are acidic and potentially cause rashes. A bit of lemon or lime juice in water or food shouldn't cause any problems.
- Shellfish is highly allergenic, so if there are allergies in the family, avoid it.
- Nuts are potential allergens, but you must assess your family's potential.

See Chapter 7 for more information.

TIPPING THE SCALE: SOLIDS AND WEIGHT GAIN

Sometimes a baby's weight doesn't increase as quickly as your doctor might like to see, according to the growth charts you see at each visit. However, most of the charts are based on formula-fed babies, so if you're breastfeeding, your baby may be in the lower percentiles on the chart. It's more important that your baby follow her own trajectory, whether breastfed or formula fed. Some babies are on the leaner side and some on the bigger side. I haven't seen any correlation between a big baby and an overweight child.

I find that these charts cause a lot of stress, but if your baby drops in his percentile, don't panic. There's often only a pound difference in the percentiles, so they really aren't the best measure of your baby's overall health. Genetics play a part in the size and weight of your baby, and development also should be taken into account. If you have an early crawler who's tearing around the house (OK, maybe this is a slight exaggeration), calories are being used up faster than in a baby who hasn't started moving yet. Maybe he's just had a growth spurt and shot up a centimetre or two, so the ratio of height to weight has changed. There are many factors to think about here.

To give you an example, I know an almost-six-year-old girl who now weighs about 45 pounds, an average weight for her age. She was born at 8 pounds, 9 ounces, and at four months had just about doubled her weight to 18 pounds, 9 ounces. By six months she was 20 pounds, and by nine months, 20 pounds, 9 ounces (yes, weight can plateau around nine to twelve months). For most of her life, up until today, her weight was off the charts at the doctors. She was exclusively breastfed until seven months, when she started on solids. No one was worried except her mom, who had to dress her in clothes for eighteen-month-olds at nine months and carry her around all day long. At one year she weighed 23 pounds, 5 ounces, at 18 months, 25 pounds, and at five years, 40 pounds. Now she is a completely average weight for her age. She levelled out and is doing just fine.

If your baby genuinely needs to put on a few extra pounds, be sure to include some higher-fat foods, which provide nine calories per gram as opposed to the four calories per gram provided by protein and carbohydrate foods. Avocado, egg yolk, olive oil, and flax oil are all healthy higher-fat foods. Coconut milk can be added to purées to provide extra fat (it's not considered a tree nut, by the way).[85]

I've heard butter and cream suggested as fatty foods to introduce, but dairy has high allergic or sensitizing potential, so it may not be the right choice for your baby. Feeding more regularly, at least three times a day, including the higher-fat foods listed above, can also quickly increase weight. If your baby was light at birth, he'll most likely catch up with his weight before you get to the point of starting solids, so it may not be necessary to keep up the higher calorie intake if the weight is increasing within his own chart. Your doctor should be consulted about all weight concerns.

FIRST FOODS CHECKLIST

Use the following checklist when introducing fruits and vegetables to your baby. I recommend starting with butternut squash and then pear, as they have the perfect texture and flavour. After that, you can alternate between any of the vegetables and fruits listed below, testing every new food for five days. See Chapter 8 for everything you need to know about making the best food for your baby.

Food	Date first given	Liked	Not too sure	Disliked	Tried again
VEGETABLES					
Butternut squash					
Sweet potato					
Broccoli					
Cauliflower					
Carrots					
Zucchini					
Parsnips					
Green beans					
Beets					
Green peas					
Turnip					

Food	Date first given	Liked	Not too sure	Disliked	Tried again
FRUITS					
Pear					
Apple					
Avocado					
Banana					
Dried apricot					
Blueberry					
Plum					
Apricot					
Papaya					
Mango					
Nectarine					

Here's another chart that you might find helpful to track what's happening with the introduction of solids.

Baby Feeding Calendar

	Sunday	Monday	Tuesday	Wednesday	Thursday	Friday	Saturday
Milk (mL/time):							
Food:							
Reactions:							
Poo:							
Other (teething/vaccinations/sickness):							

Milk: How many mL of formula or length of time if breastfed?

Food: What did baby eat, how much, and at what time?

Reactions: Anything from rashes anywhere on the body to runny nose, constipation, diarrhea, gassiness, bloating, etc.

Poo: How many? Describe.

Other (teething/vaccinations/sickness): Anything else going on that may contribute to symptoms.

RECIPES FOR 6- TO 9-MONTH-OLDS

For years, participants in my Mommy Chef cooking classes have followed these first foods recipes with great success. I hope you'll find them helpful, too. Remember, go slow and steady—this isn't a race!

Try to buy as much organic produce as you can. See "The Shopper's Guide to Pesticides" on page 149 for most important fruits and veggies to buy organic.

Note: The quantities below are approximate, as fruit and vegetable sizes vary. Water added to purées should be filtered with a Brita or reverse osmosis. Unless otherwise stated, all purées can be stored in the refrigerator for up to three days, and in the freezer, up to three months.

BUTTERNUT SQUASH PURÉE

I recommend this as a first food—babies love the smooth texture and flavour, and it's sweet but not too sweet.

1 lb	butternut squash	500 g

1. Peel, deseed, and chop squash into small cubes.
2. Steam until tender, about 15 to 20 minutes.
3. Purée, adding ½ to 1 cup (125 to 250 mL) water, until it reaches the texture of a smooth, thick soup. Makes about 3 cups (750 mL).

Note: Squash tends to be a little watery after defrosting, so make this purée slightly thicker if you're going to freeze it.

NUTRITIONAL INFORMATION
Butternut squash is a good source of vitamin A (in the form of beta carotene), vitamin C, potassium, fibre, manganese, folic acid, vitamins B1, B3, and B6, copper, and pantothenic acid.

Pear Purée

Pear is a lovely second food to introduce. Smooth and sweet, it's a common favourite!

8	pears (D'Anjou, Bartlett, or Bosc)	8

1. Peel, core, and chop pears into medium-sized cubes.
2. Steam until tender, about 7 to 10 minutes.
3. Purée until smooth (no added water needed). Makes about 3 cups (750 mL).

NUTRITIONAL INFORMATION
Pears are a good source of vitamin C and fibre.

Blueberry Purée

Don't be afraid to serve your baby this purée, even though it can be messy! Keep in mind, it does have a little texture from the skins, so it might be best to wait until four or more foods are introduced. Expect blueberry poo to change to a dark colour as well.

2 ½ cups	frozen or fresh wild blueberries	625 mL

1. Steam blueberries until just heated through, about 5 to 7 minutes.
2. Purée until smooth, about 5 minutes, adding ½ to 1 cup (125 to 250 mL) water, depending on how much has come out of the blueberries while steaming. Makes about 2 ½ cups (575 mL).

NUTRITIONAL INFORMATION
Blueberries are high in antioxidants and a good source of vitamin C, manganese, fibre, and vitamin E.

Banana Purée

Banana is a well-loved fruit and so easy to prepare. When you're out and about and stuck for something to feed your baby, find a banana, mash, and serve.

1	ripe banana	1

1. Peel and mash banana with a fork or the back of a spoon. Stir in breast milk or formula to desired consistency. Makes about ½ cup (125 mL).

NUTRITIONAL INFORMATION
Bananas are a good source of vitamin B6, vitamin C, potassium, dietary fibre, and manganese.

Avocado Purée

Avocado is a powerhouse of nutrients and monounsaturated fat. An amazing food for putting on extra weight if your baby needs it, but don't shy away from it if she doesn't.

¼ to ½	ripe avocado	¼ to ½

1. Remove the pit from the avocado and scoop out the flesh with a spoon. Mash with a fork or the back of a spoon until smooth. Stir in breast milk or formula if necessary to desired consistency. Serve immediately. Not suitable for freezing. Makes 2 to 4 tablespoons (25 to 60 mL).

NUTRITIONAL INFORMATION
Avocados are a good source of vitamin K, fibre, vitamin B6, vitamin C, folate, copper, and potassium.

SWEET POTATO PURÉE

Babies seem to love the orange vegetables, and this one's definitely a favourite. Sweet potatoes are high in fibre so you'll need to add lots of water to thin it and help the fibre move through baby's digestive system. Try adding ½ teaspoon cinnamon next time you make a batch.

2	medium sweet potatoes or yams	2

1. Peel and chop sweet potato into small cubes.
2. Steam until tender, about 15 to 20 minutes.
3. Purée, adding 1 ¾ to 2 ½ cups (400 to 625 mL) water until it reaches the texture of a smooth, thick soup. Makes about 4 cups (1 L).

Note: Sweet potato tends to be a little watery after defrosting, so make this purée slightly thicker if you're going to freeze it.

NUTRITIONAL INFORMATION
Sweet potatoes are a good source of beta carotene, fibre, potassium, and vitamins C and E.

APPLE PURÉE

Apple purée, or applesauce, is one dish that you'll be making for a long time! It's a firm favourite from the baby stage well into adulthood.

8	apples (Fuji, Gala, or Pink Lady)	8

1. Peel, core, and chop apples into small cubes.
2. Steam until tender, about 10 minutes.
3. Purée, adding ¼ to ½ cup (50 to 125 mL) water until it reaches the texture of a smooth, thick soup. Makes about 3 cups (750 mL).

NUTRITIONAL INFORMATION
Apples are a good source of fibre, vitamin C, and flavonoids.

Broccoli Purée

Many parents worry that broccoli will give their babies gas, but that's not necessarily the case. As with any other food, try it and watch for reaction.

1 head	broccoli	1 head

1. Peel broccoli stem to remove fibrous outer layer and cut about 1 inch (2.5 cm) off the bottom and discard. Chop broccoli florets and stem into small pieces.
2. Steam until tender, about 10 to 15 minutes.
3. Purée, adding ¼ to ½ cup (125 to 150 mL) water until it reaches the texture of a smooth, thick soup. Makes about 3 cups (750 mL).

NUTRITIONAL INFORMATION
Broccoli is a good source of calcium, magnesium, beta carotene, folic acid, potassium, and vitamin C.

Cauliflower Purée

Cauliflower's delicate, creamy taste lends itself to many combinations of purée. On the odd occasion I've seen babies become gassy with cauliflower, but not as often as you might think!

1 head	cauliflower	1 head

1. Remove core and stem from cauliflower. Chop florets into small pieces.
2. Steam until tender, about 15 minutes.
3. Purée, adding ¼ to ½ cup (125 to 150 mL) water until it reaches the texture of a smooth, thick soup. Makes about 3 cups (750 mL).

NUTRITIONAL INFORMATION
Steamed cauliflower is a good source of vitamin C, folate, fibre, vitamin B5, vitamin B6, and manganese.

DRIED APRICOT PURÉE

Buy organic brown and unsulphured dried apricots—they're brown because they don't contain sulphites, which can trigger asthma and gas (bright orange apricots contain sulphites). Dried apricots have a laxative effect, so they're great for treating constipation. This purée is very sweet.

1 cup	dried apricots (unsulphured)	250 mL

1. Put apricots into a saucepan and cover with filtered water. Simmer until plump and softened, about 10 minutes.
2. Transfer all contents, including any remaining water, to a bowl; purée until it reaches the texture of a smooth, thick soup. If you're freezing the purée, you might need to add an extra ¼ cup (50 mL) water for it to freeze solid.
3. Serve alone or combine with pears, papaya, avocado, or any other fruit favourite. Makes about 3 cups (750 mL).

NUTRITIONAL INFORMATION
Apricots are a good source of beta carotene, potassium, iron, calcium, silicon, phosphorus, and vitamin C. The copper and cobalt in apricots is beneficial in treating anemia. In some animal studies, dried apricots were just as effective as liver, kidneys, or eggs in treating iron-deficiency anemia. Ounce for ounce compared to fresh, dried apricots contain twelve times as much iron, seven times the fibre, and five times the vitamin A!

ZUCCHINI (SUMMER SQUASH) PURÉE

A simple yet delectable purée that's fast to make!

2	large zucchini	2

1. Trim the ends off the zucchini and chop into small cubes.
2. Steam gently until tender, about 5 to 10 minutes.
3. Purée until smooth (no water needed). Makes about 3 cups (750 mL).

NUTRITIONAL INFORMATION
Zucchini is a good source of manganese, vitamin C, magnesium, vitamin A, fibre, potassium, copper, folate, and phosphorus.

Carrot Purée

Carrots are well liked for their sweet flavour.

10	medium carrots	10

1. Peel and chop carrots into small cubes.
2. Steam until tender, about 20 minutes.
3. Purée, adding ½ to 1 cup (125 to 250 mL) water until it reaches the texture of a smooth, thick soup. Makes about 3 cups (750 mL).

NUTRITIONAL INFORMATION
Carrots are a good source of beta carotene and fibre.

Parsnip Purée

Babies love this smooth, creamy purée. I constantly hear, "I've never tried a parsnip before" from moms in my Mommy Chef cooking classes. Now's your chance!

5 to 6	medium parsnips	5 to 6

1. Peel and chop parsnips into small cubes.
2. Steam until tender, about 10 to 15 minutes.
3. Purée to desired consistency, adding 1 ½ to 2 cups (375 to 500 mL) water until it reaches the texture of a smooth, thick soup. Makes about 3 cups (750 mL).

NUTRITIONAL INFORMATION
Parsnips are a good source of fibre, calcium, iron, potassium, some B vitamins, and vitamin C.

BEETROOT PURÉE

A good source of iron, beets have a lovely sweet but earthy flavour. If your baby isn't sure about the taste, try beets again as a finger food at 9 to 12 months.

2	large, fresh beets	2

1. Peel and chop beets into very small pieces.
2. Steam until tender, about 45 minutes. Purée, adding ½ to 1 cup (150 to 250 mL) water until it reaches the texture of a smooth, thick soup. Makes about 3 cups (750 mL).

NUTRITIONAL INFORMATION
Beets are a good source of folic acid, manganese, potassium, fibre, vitamin C, magnesium, iron, copper, and phosphorus.

PLUM PURÉE

The dark pigment of plums lets you know that they're high in antioxidants. This luscious purée is a treat for anyone. If the plums are too tart, stir in some apple or pear purée.

10	ripe plums	10

1. Slice plums in half vertically, and twist to reveal and remove the pits (no peeling required). Cut into quarters.
2. Steam until tender, about 10 minutes.
3. Purée, adding water if necessary. Makes about 3 cups (750 mL).

NUTRITIONAL INFORMATION
Plums are a good source of vitamin C, vitamin A, vitamin B2, potassium, and fibre.

FRESH APRICOT PURÉE

A treat in the summer when apricots are fresh. Apricots are on the list of fruits to buy organic.

10	ripe apricots	10

1. Slice apricots in half vertically, and twist to reveal and remove the pits. Cut into quarters.
2. Steam until tender, about 10 minutes.
3. Purée, adding water if necessary, until it reaches the texture of a smooth, thick soup. Makes about 3 cups (750 mL).

NUTRITIONAL INFORMATION
Apricots are an excellent source of vitamin A, vitamin C, fibre, and potassium.

GREEN BEAN PURÉE

You can make this with both green and yellow beans.

1 ½ lb	green beans	750 g

1. Trim the stem ends and chop the beans into ³/₄-inch (2 cm) pieces.
2. Steam until tender, about 5 to 10 minutes.
3. Purée with ¼ to ½ cup (125 to 150 mL) water until it reaches the texture of a smooth, thick soup. Makes about 3 cups (750 mL).

NUTRITIONAL INFORMATION
Green beans are a good source of vitamin C, vitamin K, manganese, vitamin A, fibre, potassium, folate, and iron.

ASPARAGUS PURÉE

Asparagus is a nutritious spring vegetable that can be purchased conventional (not organic)—bugs don't like them, so they don't need to be sprayed much, if at all.

12	asparagus spears	12

1. Chop 3/4 inch (2 cm) off the bottom of the spear, or snap off the woody ends, and discard. Chop into 3/4 inch (2 cm pieces).
2. Steam until tender, about 5 to 7 minutes.
3. Purée with 2 to 3 tablespoons (25 to 50 mL) water until it reaches the texture of a smooth, thick soup. Makes about 3 cups (750 mL).

NUTRITIONAL INFORMATION
Asparagus is a good source of vitamin A, vitamin C, potassium, folic acid, zinc, and fibre.

PEA AND MINT PURÉE

Mint perfectly complements the peas and adds unexpected zip.

1	carrot	1
1 ½ cups	fresh or frozen peas	375 mL
¼ tsp	chopped fresh mint	1 mL

1. Peel and chop carrot into small cubes and steam for about 15 minutes. Add peas and steam until tender, about 5 to 10 minutes longer.
2. Purée with mint and enough water to reach the texture of a smooth, thick soup. Makes about 1 ½ cups (375 mL).

NUTRITIONAL INFORMATION
Green peas are a good source of vitamin C, vitamin K, manganese, fibre, folate, thiamine (vitamin B1), and iron.

PEAR AND APPLE PURÉE

Scrumptious purée!

4	medium apples (Gala, Fuji, or Pink Lady)	4	
4	medium pears (D'Anjou, Bartlett, or Bosc)	4	

1. Peel, core, and chop apples and pears into small cubes.
2. Steam until tender, about 15 minutes.
3. Purée, adding a little water, until it reaches the texture of a smooth, thick soup. Makes about 3 cups (750 mL).

NUTRITIONAL INFORMATION
A good source of fibre, vitamin C, and flavonoids.

AVOCADO AND PEAR PURÉE

Creamy and delicious, avocado is a good source of nutritious fat to add to any purée. You can add some raw garlic before mashing if baby is getting sick—it's a great way to boost the immune system.

¼	avocado	¼	
¼	pear*	¼	

1. Remove the pit from the avocado and scoop out the flesh with a spoon. Peel the pear.
2. Mash together or use your hand blender or chopper. Serve immediately. Makes about 1 cup (250 mL).

* Papaya or banana can be used as well as or instead of pear. Next time add some blueberries.

NUTRITIONAL INFORMATION
Avocados are a good source of vitamin K, fibre, vitamin B6, vitamin C, folate, copper, and potassium.

CARROT AND APPLE PURÉE

This is a simple dish that's high in antioxidants.

4	medium carrots	4
4	apples (Gala, Fuji, or Pink Lady)	4

1. Peel and chop carrots into small cubes. Steam for about 15 minutes.
2. Peel, core, and chop apples into 1-inch (2.5 cm) chunks and add to carrots. Steam until tender, about 10 minutes longer.
3. Purée, adding enough water to reach the texture of a smooth, thick soup. Makes about 3 cups (750 mL).

NUTRITIONAL INFORMATION
A good source of vitamin A, vitamin C, vitamin K, fibre, and potassium.

BUTTERNUT SQUASH AND PEAR PURÉE

Your baby will love this wonderful combination. Try sprinkling it with a bit of cinnamon, too.

1 lb	butternut squash	500 g
1	very ripe pear	1

1. Peel, seed, and chop butternut squash into small cubes. Steam for about 10 minutes.
2. Peel, core, and chop pear into small cubes and add to steamer. Steam until tender, about 5 minutes longer.
3. Mash or purée with a hand blender, adding water if necessary.

NUTRITIONAL INFORMATION
A good source of beta carotene, vitamin C, potassium, fibre, and manganese.

BEET AND APPLE PURÉE

You can substitute parsnip for the apples to make a lovely smooth, pink purée!

1	large, fresh beet	1
4	apples (Gala, Fuji, or Pink Lady)	4

1. Peel and chop beets into very small cubes. Steam for about 40 minutes.
2. Peel, core, and chop apples and add to steamer. Steam until tender, about 10 minutes longer.
3. Purée, adding enough water to reach the texture of a smooth, thick soup. Makes about 3 cups (750 mL).

NUTRITIONAL INFORMATION
A good source of vitamin C, folic acid, manganese, potassium, magnesium, iron, copper, and phosphorus.

CARROT AND PARSNIP PURÉE

Carrots and parsnips are a wonderful combination that your baby is sure to enjoy.

5	medium carrots	5
2	medium parsnips	2

1. Peel and chop carrots into small cubes. Steam for about 10 minutes.
2. Peel and chop parsnips and add to steamer. Steam until tender, about 15 minutes longer.
3. Purée, adding enough water to reach the texture of a smooth, thick soup. Makes about 3 cups (750 mL).

NUTRITIONAL INFORMATION
A good source of vitamin A, vitamin C, vitamin K, fibre, calcium, iron, potassium, and some B vitamins.

PLUM AND PEAR PURÉE

This fast, fresh purée is packed with vitamins, antioxidants, and fibre. Tart plums and sweet pears combine wonderfully.

4	ripe plums	4
2	pears	2

1. Cut the plums in half and remove the pits. Peel and core the pears. Cut the fruit into small pieces.
2. Steam until tender, about 5 minutes.
3. Purée in a food processor or with a hand blender, adding a little water to reach the texture of a smooth, thick soup. Older babies can eat it chunky and with a pinch of cinnamon. Makes about 3 cups (750 mL).

NUTRITIONAL INFORMATION
A good source of vitamin C, vitamin A, vitamin B2, potassium, and fibre.

WATERMELON, PEACH, AND BASIL PURÉE

This refreshing "raw" purée is packed with enzymes and nutrients.

2 ½ cups	seedless watermelon	625 mL
2 cups	peaches	500 mL
¼ tsp	chopped fresh basil or mint	1 mL

1. Remove the pits from the peaches and cut the fruit into small pieces.
2. Purée with basil in a food processor or with a hand blender, until smooth. Makes about 5 cups (1.25 L).

NUTRITIONAL INFORMATION
A good source of vitamin C, vitamin A, vitamin B6, thiamine, potassium, and magnesium.

OAT CEREAL

If you choose to give your baby cereal, I recommend oats, as they're the least allergenic and are naturally high in both soluble and insoluble fibre, as well as iron.

1 cup	oats*	250 mL

1. Grind oats in a coffee grinder to a fine powder. Store in an airtight container.
2. To make cereal, pour ¼ cup (75 mL) water into a saucepan and bring to a boil.
3. Slowly add 1 tablespoon (15 mL) ground oats while whisking vigorously. Reduce heat and simmer for about 10 minutes.
4. Set aside to cool and stir in your baby's favourite fruit purée (apple, pear, and apricot are good) for natural sweetness and a nutrient boost. You can also thin it with breast milk or formula. Makes about 2 tablespoons (30 mL) cereal without the fruit purée.

*Steel-cut oats are preferable but have more texture.

NUTRITIONAL INFORMATION
Oats are a good source of manganese, selenium, iron, vitamin B1, fibre, magnesium, protein, and phosphorus.

INTRODUCTION OF SOLIDS SCHEDULE

This is a general guideline to follow from the introduction of solids to the time when your baby's eating three meals a day, usually by nine months. But don't worry if your baby isn't following this order exactly—every baby is different, and this table is intended just to give you an example of how to introduce solids and progress. Start with either lunch or dinner (this table shows lunch).

Introduction of Solids:	Upon Rising	Breakfast	Sleep	Lunch	Sleep	Dinner	Bedtime
First 3 to 4 weeks	Milk*		Milk	Milk and half an hour later, solid food To progress, increase the number of cubes in a feeding	Milk	Milk	Milk
Next 3 to 4 weeks	Milk	Milk	Milk	Milk and solids	Milk	Milk and half an hour later, introduce the second meal To progress, increase the number of cubes in a feeding	Milk
From about 8 to 9 months onward	Milk	Milk and half an hour later, introduce the third meal To progress, increase the number of cubes in a feeding	Milk	Milk and solids	Milk	Milk and solids	Milk

* "Milk" is either breast milk or formula.

THE NEXT STAGE
9- to 12-Month Chunkier Meals

By now, your baby ideally will have been enjoying a great repertoire of fruits and vegetables. That's the perfect picture, but it doesn't always go that way. However, with any luck you've been able to offer the following yummy and nutritious foods: butternut squash, sweet potato, broccoli, cauliflower, zucchini, carrots, parsnips, green beans, beets, pear, apple, avocado, banana, dried apricots, blueberries, plums, apricots, papaya, and nectarine. Your baby may have tried other foods than those listed here, or if he's moving at his own speed, he might not have made it through all these foods. Every baby is unique and will move along in his own time, and although that pace may not be what you had in mind, it's probably right for him. If there's anything on the above list that you haven't tried, go for it. It's always great to expose your baby to new foods and flavours.

WHAT TO DO AFTER PURÉE

It's time to start thinking about chunkier meals and finger foods. Starting on purées with more texture may be daunting, but you won't know how your baby handles it until you try. There's no rush for this next stage. Try to purée your food a bit less, leaving some chunks, lumps, or bumps in your scrumptious creation. If feeding goes well, then less puréeing of some foods is the new way forward. But keep offering smooth purées as well, to vary the textures. If your baby still gags with the slightest chunk, try again in another week, as the gag reflex needs to relax before lumpier food can pass.

Around 9 months of age, new independence and skills bring a whole new meaning to mealtimes. Your baby may want to start practising the pincer grip (first finger and thumb coming together) by picking up small pieces of food, objects, or even the smallest bit of fluff on the floor that you need a magnifying glass to see. Offering small pieces of food to practise hand–eye coordination and the pincer grip is lots of fun but can lead to a great big mess. But baby needs a lot of practice to master this new skill. Not all babies start with the pincer grip at 9 months—some begin at 8 months, others closer to 10 months. Some

> ### Help for Gagging
> Osteopathy can help with the premature or hyperactive gag reflex, which may have something to do with a forceps birth. If your baby has a really hard time swallowing lumps or bumps without gagging, find your nearest osteopath, see if she treats babies and children, and make an appointment. Although I prefer that babies eat purées (though not always smooth) for a long time, as you can get more nutrients into them, having a strong reflex that leads to throwing up the whole meal isn't to their benefit. Osteopathy is a gentle, hands-on treatment that aims to release restriction and constriction so that normal function can resume.

babies start with the full hand pickup when they grab at some food on their plate or tray and try to get it into their mouths, with or without opening their hands (it's good for a laugh, that's for sure!). As baby gets older and these skills become more precise, she learns how to open her hand to grasp the food in a full hand pickup—an important new understanding.

Most parents worry about their baby choking on chunkier and finger foods, to the point where they might put off offering them. Choking is rare and not to be mixed up with gagging, which is very normal. Usually, this is when parents think about signing up for first aid training, including what to do in the case of choking—essential information for every parent. Now that you know what to do, you can offer new foods with a bit more confidence. There are certain foods that I would suggest staying away from until your baby is much older, including small, round foods such as whole grapes (cut them into small pieces until they're 12 to 18 months old, and then just be mindful), but fear shouldn't stop you from allowing your baby to move toward chunkier and finger foods. Everyone needs to gain confidence when it comes to starting on finger foods, both parents and baby. Gagging, the thrusting of food from the back of the throat forward into the mouth, is an important reflex to keep your baby from harm. And it works well in most circumstances, protecting your baby from a food she's not ready for.

FINGER FOODS

Start slowly with finger foods. Putting finger foods on the high chair tray after a meal is a great way to start. Try placing a 1/4-inch (5 mm) well-steamed piece of carrot, halved or quartered, in baby's mouth and see what happens. Steamed cauliflower pieces melt in the mouth (try it first yourself), so this is another good one to try. Some parents get very excited about self-feeding, but I caution you about moving forward with too much independence, as I commonly see the refusal of purée when finger foods begin. Some babies are more independent and want to feed themselves but can't self-feed with a spoon yet. The problem arises when their food consumption drops because there's only so much they can feed themselves at one sitting. You can also get a better variety of foods into a purée than on the high chair tray. I commonly see a drop in weight and a change in overall eating habits with this scenario, usually not for the better. Parents sometimes worry that their baby isn't getting what he needs because of the limited number of foods that can be made into finger foods, and all sorts of new foods, including toast and cheese, then become a staple. It's very difficult to get leafy greens into anything other than a purée at this stage. So do what you can to keep purée part of most meals for as long as you can—offer his main meal of purée first, then a few pieces of finger food to play with afterward. Although there seems to be some mysterious pressure to steer your baby away from purée on to table foods, I'd rather see one-year-olds eating textured purées or soft foods, such as noodles, mixed with a rainbow of colours. Purée is also the perfect place to hide those fruits or vegetables that offer fantastic nutrition but are not well loved.

Another aspect to finger feeding is that it can be messy—food ends up all over baby, on the floor, or all over you, and you might feel that you're the one who needs the bib. Try to get over the need to be clean while eating. Feeling what happens to a handful of steamed broccoli when it's scooped up into a little hand and squished is good for the tactile senses. Clean her up at the end, or have the bath ready for a full body wash.

My daughter loved frozen wild organic blueberries. She had a great pincer grip and would eat about half a cup of them, frozen, every morning for about a year. But when we went on a trip to England when she was 15 months old, we couldn't find them anywhere. I suddenly realized that her little fingernails were constantly stained from the blueberries, because when she didn't have them, her hands looked clean again. I had gotten so used to her purple fingers that I didn't notice them anymore!

Just because your baby is into finger foods doesn't mean that you need to abandon the great fruits and vegetables you've been offering up until now. A lot of the vegetables that your baby has been enjoying can be steamed, chopped into small pieces (but not so small that they're difficult to pick up), and given as part of the meal. Make batches of finger food, as you did with your purée, and freeze them in ice cube trays or on a baking tray before putting them in freezer bags. Grab a handful, defrost overnight in the fridge, or drop them into boiling water for a few minutes, and serve with the meal.

This is the stage when avoiding cereals and grains becomes trickier, with peer pressure to give off-the-shelf foods that a friend's baby loves. But toast, bread, and other refined starches fill your baby up on less nutrient-dense foods that can be hard to digest because he's not yet producing enough of the digestive enzyme amylase at full strength.

My best tip at this stage is to stay out of the baby aisles at the supermarket. Foods that are marketed for babies are not necessarily the healthiest. One of the oldest baby cookies, Farley's Rusks, were first made in the United Kingdom by Heinz and are well known in other countries. A recent article published in *The Times* newspaper in England commented that the original biscuit "contains more sugar than McVitie's dark chocolate digestives," a cookie coated on one side with chocolate.[86] Baby Mum Mums are another popular, well-marketed baby cracker available in Canada. The original rice rusks, as they're sometimes called, are made of japonica rice, sugar, skim milk powder, and salt. Just pause and think about those ingredients for a moment. *White rice, sugar, milk, and salt.* Who ever advised that they were appropriate for a baby? I believe that any doctor or dentist would agree that these ingredients are not beneficial for anyone—let alone your baby! The company's website suggests that Mum Mums are suitable for babies who are ready for solids. I have to completely, wholeheartedly disagree with every ingredient in this product. First of all, salt should be avoided until at least a year of age, as it's too taxing on little kidneys. Two conveniently wrapped crackers contain 15 g sodium, along with 15 calories, 4 g carbohydrates, and 0.3 g protein, but 0 percent of the daily recommended value of vitamin A, vitamin C, calcium, and iron.[87] For exclusively breastfed babies, offering skim milk powder may cause rashes, gassiness, diarrhea, or constipation, to name a few possibilities, not to mention the increased potential for allergies (see Chapter 7). Even formula-fed babies may react because the milk powder is unhydrolyzed (or not broken down). Dairy sensitivity can cause eczema to flare up. And although most parents consciously avoid giving sugar to their babies, one serving not only increases your baby's blood sugar levels, but also suppresses the effectiveness of the immune system and leaves a trail of sugar all over those new baby teeth that may have just broken through (an opportune time for bacteria to thrive). I have yet to see a parent with a toothbrush in hand after baby polishes off one or two of these crackers. In recent years, a few new varieties have hit the market, including organic original, vegetable, and organic Toddler Mum Mums, some without the skim milk powder, but with more sugar and salt added. The nutritional profile of the organic Mum Mums is comparable to the same quantity of Rice Krispy Square. If I offered you a piece of a Rice Krispy Square, would you give it to your baby? I think not. Whenever I bring up this product in a workshop or Mommy Chef class, I always hear, "But my baby loves them." No wonder—babies have a natural sweet tooth, and unfortunately, they don't know well enough to say, "No thanks, Mom."

Sugar and the Immune System

Sugar slows down the ability to fight off infections, so it's best to avoid it when your baby has a cold or is teething, if not all the time as prevention. When white blood cells are exposed to high levels of sugar in the bloodstream, they are less able to engulf bacteria and have weakened systemic resistance to all infections. So it's a good idea to limit sugar every day, particularly while your baby is showing signs of illness such as a cold or flu. You might think that giving a teething biscuit while a tooth is coming in will help your baby, but in actual fact, the sugar in the biscuit slows down the immune army further (it's already busy thinking that an erupting tooth is something to defend against).

It's your job to read ingredient lists—not only the nutritional composition, but also what's actually in the product you're about to purchase for your baby. Other teething biscuits found in the baby aisle have honey (not to be given until one year, remember), wheat (very aggravating to the digestive system), salt, sugar, high levels of saturated fat, and no real nutrients to speak of. Your baby's stomach is only so big, and you want to fill it with it nutritious food that will support her development and growth, not slow it down.

So if you're to stay out of the baby aisle in the supermarket, which finger foods are nutritious and safe? I've listed some suggestions below, with explanations so you'll know which foods are nutritious and which may be more useful for giving baby practice with his new skills. Remember: When you're introducing a new food, try to wait four days before offering another one. Maintaining this practice can get complicated at this stage, but if you don't, this might be the one time that you see a reaction and you won't know where it came from.

FINGER FOOD SUGGESTIONS

Aim for as much organic food as possible without any added refined sugar.

- Soft, ripe fruit, cut up or bitten by you into small pieces.
- Small pieces of grapes (I peeled some of the skin off with my teeth the first few times as it made my daughter gag) or champagne grapes (these are very small and are available in the summer).
- Small pieces of ripe pear (no skin), apples (no skin, and be careful as it's a hard fruit), melon, plum, peach, mango, papaya, raspberries, banana, and apricots.
- Frozen organic wild blueberries (smaller than nonwild), a big hit that's packed with antioxidants and is one of nature's superfoods. Keep them frozen so they're not quite as messy; frozen berries also feel great on sore gums.
- Steamed and cut-up veggies: green beans, sweet potato, asparagus, broccoli, carrots, beets, peas, cauliflower, corn, and parsnips.
- Cut-up dried fruit: apple, apricots, and raisins. Dried fruit is very high in iron and makes an excellent snack. It has some texture, so encourage chewing even if baby doesn't have teeth yet (the gums are quite powerful)—otherwise, you may find undigested raisins in the diaper. Dried fruit also needs to be broken down with the gums or teeth to get the nutritional benefit. If you find that your

raisins are too hard, soak them in boiling water for a few minutes to soften, and cool before serving. As your baby gets more teeth, be sure to give them a wipe or brush after eating dried fruit, as it can stick between or in premolars or molars and cause cavities.

- Peas and beans: chickpeas (garbanzo beans), black-eyed peas, adzuki, cannellini, kidney, black, navy, pinto, mung, and borlotti. Start slowly with these as they pose a choking hazard, and remove the skin from chickpeas so baby doesn't choke on it. Squish with your fingers or mash with a fork to serve, offering small pieces to start. Eventually, your baby will get the hang of round foods like green peas and enjoy them whole without any help.

The following recommendations are for cereal products that are gluten free, sugar free, and dairy free.

- Rice Puff Cereal (Nature's Path)—not rice crisps but puffs (organic, whole grain, and sugar free). I call this the novice picker-upper food. They melt in the mouth easily and are big enough to practise the pincer grip with. Nutritional value is limited, but they're a great practice tool.
- Millet Puff Cereal (Nature's Path). Excellent for giving purée more texture, so add it to any purée to increase its texture. The puffs don't lose their shape when added to food, either. They're a bit too small to pick up with the fingers, but good to keep your little one busy practising while you make dinner.
- Rice cakes (brown rice, salt free, and organic). Start by breaking off small pieces to eat, and then as confidence grows, give half and then whole cakes. Try to find thin rice cakes at health food stores. Again, they're not to be relied on for great nutritional value, but you can spread them with hummus or almond butter or even make a rice cake sandwich with apple butter or fruit juice–sweetened fruit spread, a healthier jam.
- Short-grain brown organic rice. There's a lot of texture here, so start by mixing with a vegetable-rich purée; closer to 10 to 12 months, the rice alone can be put on baby's tray. Provides great nutrients, including B vitamins, iron, and fibre. Short-grain tends to be a bit stickier than long-grain rice, so it's easier for little fingers to pick up.
- Barbara's O Cereal—a healthier alternative to other "o" products. It's organic, low in salt, and sweetened with fruit juice, not sugar. Melts in the mouth easily, but I would say that this is a stage-two finger food for those who are hesitant.

- Noodles made from brown rice, quinoa, or amaranth. Start with a penne or elbow macaroni and cut up the tubes into smaller pieces. These can be added to a purée (my favourite is Introduction to Lentils at the end of this chapter) or served plain as a finger food.

NEW FOODS ON THE MENU

As your baby grows, his digestive system continues to mature, and he may be ready now to digest some new foods as well as handle more texture. You might feel a bit bored with your menu options of simple fruits and vegetables, so here are a few new foods to jazz up mealtime.

Legumes and beans such as chickpeas; kidney, adzuki, cannellini, and mung beans; split peas; and lentils can be introduced. This opens up a whole new world of possibilities. Red lentils are fantastic added to any purée at this stage. Cooking vegetables in a saucepan (as opposed to steaming) with adequate water and a handful of rinsed red lentils increases the fibre, protein, and beta carotene content of any dish. Red lentils are a great first food with texture because they don't maintain their shape as green (also known as French or du Puy) lentils do. Chickpeas cook well in purées and can be mashed to make hummus. Once chickpeas have been offered in purée, you can start to give them as a finger food.

Egg yolk is an excellent source of nutrients, including iron; zinc; calcium; magnesium; potassium; selenium; folic acid; vitamin B12; fat-soluble vitamins A, D, E, and K; essential fatty acids (from chickens fed with EFA-rich seeds); and cholesterol. The yolk has an exceptionally absorbable form of protein, second only to that found in breast milk, according to Dr. Sears.[88]

Eggs have been unfairly stigmatized as being high in cholesterol and possibly contributing to heart disease. This isn't completely true. The egg scare came about because of a study in the 1930s where people consumed large quantities of dried egg powder. This was shown to raise cholesterol. But dried egg powder contains oxidized fat, which is rancid fat, and that is what raised the cholesterol. In subsequent studies, some people have been able to eat 10 fresh hardboiled eggs a day for 30 days without their cholesterol levels going up![89] So giving egg yolk offers your baby a nutrient-packed food that's low in saturated fat.

Choose organic eggs for your baby. Conventional chickens are usually given GM feed (containing corn), which can pass into the egg and is then eaten by you or your baby. GM foods are a newish breed and have the potential to seriously affect health in a negative way. For more information, see www.responsibletechnology.org.

The first time you offer egg, be sure that you don't contaminate the yolk with the white. Boil the egg for seven to eight minutes until it's completely cooked but not dried out and chalky. Cool, separate the white from the yolk, mash, and serve. You can also try mixing the yolk with a favourite purée. Once you're sure there's no reaction, you can do an egg yolk scramble or omelette for variety of texture.

Eggs have higher allergic potential, so proceed cautiously. If your baby has had a reaction to her vaccinations, offer a very small amount at first, as she may already have developed antibodies that will produce a reaction. Avoid egg white until one year as it has an even higher allergic potential than the yolk.

The least allergenic nut and seed butters can also be introduced now. Almond butter, sesame seed butter (tahini), and sunflower seed butter are a powerhouse of essential fatty acids; minerals such as calcium, magnesium, manganese, and zinc; and fibre and protein. In the form of raw butters, they offer the full spectrum of beneficial fats, whereas the roasted or toasted butters have been heated, denaturing these good fats. Spread them or add to purées to increase nutritional content and protein.

As with eggs, nuts and seeds have a higher allergic potential. Assess your own situation—if you have a family history of allergies or your baby has eczema, for instance, proceed slowly. On first introduction, give a small amount of these butters without any other new food. I often recommend to concerned parents dabbing a bit of tahini or almond butter on their baby's cheek or inside lip and waiting to see whether a reaction develops. Look out for redness on the cheek or hives, the most common reactions, although symptoms can vary. Giving a small quantity allows the body the chance to react to a lesser degree, while ideally having a more desensitizing effect (a slow introduction of a small amount of food might reduce the reaction of the immune system). If you introduce almond, sesame, or sunflower seed butter in a controlled situation, you're better able to assess the reaction than if your baby is exposed to it without your knowledge and you have no idea where the resulting rash has come from. The next ingestion also might cause more serious symptoms.

Newer recommendations and research suggest that offering a small amount of a potentially allergenic substance may actually reduce the chances of your baby developing an allergy to that food. I'm suggesting that you give your potentially allergic child tahini when mom, dad, or siblings are allergic to sesame, but giving a little bit may help to keep nonallergic child that way—allergy free. See Chapter 7 for more on allergies.

Iron- and zinc-rich foods are important at the 9- to 12-month stage to aid in growth and maturation of tissues. Fibre, found in all fruits and vegetables, is encouraged to promote intestinal health and the colonization of good bacteria in the intestines. Daily bowel movements are essential for your baby's good health.

Both herbs and spices boast a wide variety of important nutrients, not just extra flavour. Start adding some fresh or dried herbs to your baby's food for a new taste experience: basil, oregano, rosemary, thyme, tarragon, cilantro, parsley, dill, and sage.

Spice up simple purées or fancier purées with cinnamon, coriander, cumin, curry, ginger, turmeric, paprika, and even saffron strands.

Iron-Rich Foods

- Beef, lamb, pork, chicken and turkey (especially dark meat)
- Beans, chickpeas
- Potato (with skin)
- Pumpkin
- Peas, lentils
- Sweet potatoes
- Pasta
- Whole grain bread
- Quinoa
- Dried apricots, dried peaches, figs, raisins
- Prunes and prune juice
- Nuts
- Tofu
- Blackstrap molasses
- Sunflower and pumpkin seeds

Zinc-Rich Foods

- Beef, lamb, poultry, pork, liver
- Egg yolks
- Milk products
- Fish and seafood
- Whole grains
- Beans
- Nuts
- Pumpkin seeds
- Peas, carrots, beets, cabbage (contain some zinc)

Nutrients from Spices and Herbs

Herbs

- Parsley is an excellent source of vitamins A, C, and K. It's also a good source of iron and folate.
- Cilantro helps control blood sugar, cholesterol, and free radical production. It helps stimulate digestion and is an amazing source of vitamin A, as well as lutein, which is necessary for good vision. Cilantro also contains calcium and potassium.
- Basil is an excellent source of vitamin K and a very good source of iron, calcium, and vitamin A. In addition, basil is a good source of dietary fibre, manganese, magnesium, vitamin C, and potassium.
- Oregano is a nutrient-dense herb with effective antibacterial properties. It's an excellent source of vitamin K and a very good source of iron, manganese, and dietary fibre. In addition, oregano is a good source of calcium, magnesium, vitamin A, vitamin C, and omega-3 fatty acids.
- Rosemary contains substances that are useful for stimulating the immune system, increasing circulation, and improving digestion. Rosemary also contains anti-inflammatory compounds that may make it useful for reducing the severity of asthma attacks. In addition, it's been shown to increase the blood flow to the head and brain, improving concentration. It's also a good source of the minerals iron and calcium, as well as dietary fibre. The fresh herb has 25 percent more manganese than dried rosemary (it's somehow lost in the process of drying) and 40 percent less calcium and iron, probably due to the higher water content.
- Thyme has a long history of use in natural medicine in connection with chest and respiratory problems. Thyme is an excellent source of iron, manganese, and vitamin K. It's also a very good source of calcium and a good source of dietary fibre.
- Tarragon promotes the production of bile by the liver, which aids in digestion and helps speed the process of eliminating toxic waste in the body. It offers healing properties for the stomach and liver and is reputed to be a mild sedative. Amazingly, it's extremely valuable in fighting intestinal worms.

- Dill is an antibacterial herb and offers protection against free radicals and carcinogens. Dill seed is a very good source of calcium and a good source of the minerals manganese and iron.
- Sage has been known as a memory enhancer and contains antioxidant and anti-inflammatory properties.

Spices

- Cinnamon is good for relieving nausea and vomiting, as well as diarrhea and indigestion; it also stabilizes blood sugar and has anticancer properties. Its key nutrients include calcium; iron; magnesium; phosphorus; potassium; zinc; manganese; vitamins A, B1, B2, B3, B6, and C; folate; fibre; and 12 phytochemicals (plant nutrients with powerful health benefits).
- Coriander reduces gas and colic, relieves diarrhea (especially in children), and stimulates digestion and appetite. Its key nutrients include calcium; iron; magnesium; phosphorus; potassium; zinc; manganese; vitamins A, B1, B2, B3, B6, C, and E (in leaf only); folate; fibre; and 22 phytochemicals.
- Cumin improves digestion; relieves cramping, diarrhea, gas, colic, and headaches; and is an antioxidant. Key nutrients include calcium; iron; magnesium; phosphorus; potassium; zinc; manganese; vitamins A, B1, B2, B3, B6, C, and E; folate; fibre; and 10 phytochemicals.
- Curry powder is a blend of spices that vary among different regions of the world. It's a digestive aid and appetite stimulant; it's good for treating dysentery and diarrhea; and it's antibacterial and antifungal. Key nutrients include vitamin B6, folate, calcium, magnesium, phosphorus, potassium, and copper; it's also a very good source of dietary fibre, vitamin E, vitamin K, iron, and manganese.
- Ginger alleviates nausea, morning sickness, vomiting, and motion sickness; it's antibacterial and anti-inflammatory; and it stimulates circulation, which helps relieve cramps, flatulence, dyspepsia, and colic. Key nutrients include calcium; iron; magnesium; phosphorus; potassium; zinc; manganese; vitamins A, B1, B2, B3, B6, C, and E; folate; fibre; and 22 phytochemicals.
- Turmeric is antibacterial and anti-inflammatory, increases blood circulation, decreases cholesterol, and acts as a digestive aid and liver stimulant. Key nutrients include calcium; iron; magnesium; phosphorus; potassium; zinc; copper;

manganese; selenium; vitamins B1, B2, B3, B6, and C; folate; fibre; and seven phytochemicals.

- Paprika is anti-inflammatory and immune-boosting and a powerful antioxidant. Key nutrients are vitamins A, B2, B3, B6, C, and E; calcium; iron; potassium; phosphorus; magnesium; manganese; zinc; copper; selenium, pantothenic acid; folate; fibre; and phytosterols.
- Saffron is the most expensive spice. It acts as an antioxidant, immune system stimulant, expectorant, pain reliever, and digestive aid, as well as stimulating circulation and controlling blood pressure. Key nutrients are calcium; iron; magnesium; phosphorus; potassium; zinc; manganese; selenium; vitamins A, B1, B2, B3, B6, C, and E; folate; fibre; and six phytochemicals.

DRINK UP: MOVING ON TO A SIPPY CUP

Whether a bottle has been introduced or not, this is a good time to start offering a sippy cup with water. Your baby may need a while to get the hang of a sippy cup, as it isn't as easy to get fluid out and it needs a slightly different suck than a bottle. But around nine months or even a bit before, you can start to offer the sippy cup, even if it's used only as a new chew toy. Some sippy cups have a soft, chewy top, and others, a hard one. It really doesn't matter which you offer, though your baby might find one easier than another. If the lid has a valve you can take it out, put a small amount of water in the cup, replace the lid without the valve, and slowly demonstrate the cause and effect of tipping up the cup to get the water. Once you've tried that a couple of times, put the valve back in and let your baby practise. Not only is the suck slower from a sippy cup than a bottle, but the tipping up of the cup takes some getting used to. If your baby takes a bottle already with formula or breast milk in it, keep the sippy cup for water. Some moms prefer to keep one type of vessel for specific fluids—bottle for breast milk or formula, and sippy cup for water. I wouldn't recommend the sippy cup for breast milk or formula at this stage as it tends to slow down the intake, and you don't want to discourage any "milk" drinking. It's still the main source of nutrition, even on an expanded diet of a wide variety of foods.

THE WATER DEBATE

Water is such a simple thing, or it should be. But H_2O has become as confusing as what food to start feeding your baby. Bottled, tap, distilled, spring, reverse osmosis, oxygenated, carbonated, and now vitaminized are all available to choose from. With so many options, how on earth do you decide what's best to serve your baby?

Most tap water is under strict scrutiny for any contaminants that might harm us, and local water authorities boast how clean and safe it is. In most cases, I would agree. However, if you live in a house built earlier than the 1950s, it may still have pipes soldered with lead. Across North America, there are still many lead pipes underground that are slowly being replaced. In March 2001, Dr. Richard Mass, a scientist and internationally renowned specialist in lead in water, was interviewed on CBC's *Marketplace*; the program's researchers also did their own testing for lead in tap water across Canada. They found varying levels of lead in houses built before as well as after 1970.[90] Samples are taken from water that's been flushed (or run from the tap) for three minutes. Dr. Mass suggested that this flushing eliminates the standing lead level, and the standing lead level gives a more accurate measurement. Running your tap before filling up your glass may work first thing in the morning, but this needs to happen each time you turn on the tap as 30 percent of the lead deposited in your water overnight makes its way into your tap water if it hasn't been run for 10 minutes.

There's no safe level of lead exposure for anyone, at any age. However, infants and children are most as risk because the first years are such a crucial time of development. Dr. Mass noted on *Marketplace,* "We recognize now that there is no threshold dose below which lead does not cause neurologic damage." Lead toxicity has a cumulative effect, causing neurological disorders, learning difficulties, emotional instability, aggression, decreased calcium deposition into bone, low sperm count, and sterility, as well as having an antagonistic effect on important minerals such as zinc and iron, possibly leading to anemia.

Wait times can be lengthy for having your water tested for lead, but it's important nonetheless. Contact your local water provider for further details.

Also found in tap water are apparently "safe" levels of hormones, medications, and other toxic substances. Although water authorities say that these substances are safe, this doesn't fill me with confidence since they reduced the acceptable level of lead in water after much criticism about the levels in schools. No one should be drinking any amount of someone else's medications, especially not your baby.

Chlorine is used to clean our tap water, ridding it of disease-causing bacteria and making it safe to drink. Or does it? It has solved one problem, but created another. Chlorine in tap water has been associated with asthma, eczema, and higher rates of miscarriage and birth defects. Chlorine also kills the beneficial bacteria in the gut, leading to the potential for digestive and immune problems. Bottled water and filters of all kinds have become more popular in recent years. It's worth investigating what's in your tap water and the different types of filter systems available. I recommend using at least a carbon filter to remove some chlorine and other contaminants. Brita, for instance, offers detailed information about what its filters reduce or eliminate from tap water and has a wide variety of filter options for making drinking water safer in an environmentally friendly way.

For your baby, avoid distilled water, which has no trace minerals and thus might contribute to deficiencies of certain minerals. Reverse osmosis, with an added calcium and magnesium post filter, is my preferred method of filtering water. It's safe and easy and doesn't require boiling or filtering. See the resource section for recommendations.

WATER VERSUS JUICE

Your baby needs only two type of fluids at this stage—breast milk or formula and water—which provide most of her nourishment and hydration. I strongly encourage you to avoid giving juice to your baby until absolutely necessary. That may be closer to two years of age, or sooner if your baby is dehydrated and needs extra fluids during sickness, very hot weather, or a bout of constipation, but only give a splash of juice in the sippy cup. Juice is a concentrated source of sweetness without fibre, and your baby just doesn't need it. Encourage drinking water for as long as you can. Water is needed for so many functions in the body, and one of those is energy.

RECIPES FOR 9- TO 12-MONTH-OLDS

Note: The quantities below are approximate, as fruit and vegetable sizes vary. Water added to purées should be filtered. Unless otherwise stated, all purées can be stored in the refrigerator for up to three days, and in the freezer for up to three months.

INTRODUCTION TO LENTILS

Red lentils are super easy to cook with and will keep your baby going. For toddlers, you can serve this purée as a sauce for noodles. It's wonderful on its own, mixed with rice, or served as a soup for mom and dad with extra lentils and stock.

2 cups	peeled and chopped butternut squash	500 mL
2 cups	water or no-sodium vegetable stock	500 mL
½ cup	red lentils, rinsed well	125 mL
3	carrots, peeled and chopped	3
2	stalks celery, chopped	2
1	small onion, chopped	1
1 tbsp	extra-virgin olive oil	15 mL
1 to 2 tbsp	fresh parsley, chopped (optional)	15 to 30 mL

1. Combine butternut squash, lentils, onion, carrots, celery, water or vegetable stock, and olive oil in a medium saucepan.
2. Bring to a boil, cover, and reduce heat. Simmer until vegetables are tender, about 20 minutes. Mash or purée with parsley (if using) to desired consistency. Makes about 3 cups (750 mL).

NUTRITIONAL INFORMATION
A good source of protein, beta carotene, fibre, potassium, and vitamins C and E.

CHEEKY CHICKPEAS

A hint of lemon and cilantro really makes this purée stand out!

1 ½ cups	water or no-sodium vegetable stock	375 mL
1	can (14 oz/398 mL) chickpeas, drained and rinsed	1
2	medium sweet potatoes, peeled and chopped into small cubes	2
1	small onion, finely chopped	1
2	stalks celery, chopped	2
1	carrot, peeled and chopped into small cubes	1
1 tbsp	extra-virgin olive oil	15 mL
2 tbsp	chopped fresh cilantro (or 1 tsp/5 mL dried)	30 mL
1 tsp	freshly squeezed lemon juice	5 mL

1. Combine water or vegetable stock, chickpeas, sweet potatoes, onion, celery, carrot, and olive oil in a medium saucepan.
2. Bring to a boil, cover, and reduce heat. Simmer until vegetables are tender, about 20 minutes.
3. Remove from heat and add cilantro and lemon juice. Mash or purée to desired consistency, adding water if necessary. Makes about 3 cups (750 mL).

NUTRITIONAL INFORMATION
Chickpeas, or garbanzo beans, are a good source of folate, manganese, fibre, protein, and copper.

Amazing Sweet Amaranth

This is what adults would consider a hot breakfast cereal. It's not just for babies; I still make this purée for myself—simply keep the skin on the fruit and don't purée. Delicious!

2 cups	water	500 mL
1 cup	amaranth, rinsed in a fine sieve	250 mL
2	pears, peeled, cored, and chopped	2
2	apples, peeled, cored, and chopped	2
¼ cup	frozen blueberries	50 mL
1 tsp	cinnamon	5 mL
1	½-inch (1 cm) piece ginger root, finely chopped	1

1. Combine all ingredients in a medium saucepan.
2. Bring to a boil, cover, and reduce heat to simmer, stirring often, until amaranth is tender, about 20 minutes. Purée to desired consistency. Makes about 3 cups (750 mL).

Note: Amaranth has a "sticky" texture, and care should be taken not to overcook it as it can become gummy. After this dish is frozen or refrigerated, you'll need to add more water to thin it out when reheating.

NUTRITIONAL INFORMATION
Botanically, amaranth isn't really a grain, but it has the nutritional profile of one. It surpasses whole wheat in calories, protein, iron, zinc, copper, and nearly all nutrients, and is the grain highest in folic acid, calcium, and vitamin E. Also, like wheat, amaranth is rich in the amino acid lysine. It even contains a bit of vitamin C. It also has three times as much calcium as a glass of milk!

Sweet Potato with Corn and Red Pepper

This intriguing purée is a powerhouse of nutrients, including fibre, vitamin C, and iron.

2	medium sweet potatoes, peeled and chopped into cubes	2
1 cup	fresh or frozen corn kernels	250 mL
½	red pepper, deseeded and chopped	½
1 tbsp	blackstrap molasses	15 mL

1. Steam sweet potato for about 15 minutes.
2. Add corn and chopped red pepper. Cook until vegetables are tender, about 5 minutes.
3. Transfer to a bowl and let cool. Mix in blackstrap molasses and purée or mash to desired consistency, adding water if necessary. Makes about 3 cups (750 mL).

NUTRITIONAL INFORMATION
A good source of vitamin B1, vitamin B5, folate, fibre, vitamin C, phosphorus, manganese, iron, calcium, copper, magnesium, and potassium.

Immune-Boosting Purée

This dish is incredibly popular. Vitamin C in the apples and turnip or rutabaga helps the absorption of iron from the raisins, and garlic is an incredible immune booster. A parent told me that she served this with Thanksgiving dinner and everyone loved it!

2	apples, peeled and chopped into cubes	2
1	large turnip or medium rutabaga, peeled and chopped into small cubes	1
1	parsnip, peeled and chopped into small cubes	1
1	carrot, peeled and chopped into small cubes	1
1	clove garlic, chopped	1
2 tbsp	raisins	30 mL
1 ½ cups	water	375 mL

1. Combine all ingredients in a medium saucepan.
2. Simmer for 30 to 40 minutes or until tender, adding extra water if necessary. Purée to desired consistency. Makes about 2 ½ cups (550 mL).

NUTRITIONAL INFORMATION
A good source of vitamin C, fibre, calcium, potassium, and iron.

Introducing ... Quinoa

Quinoa (kee-ne-wa) makes a savoury but sweet purée with quite a bit of texture. Set some aside before puréeing for the rest of the family to enjoy as a meal or a side dish.

2 cups	water	500 mL
1 cup	quinoa, rinsed well	250 mL
1	medium butternut squash, peeled and chopped	1
4	asparagus spears or green beans, ends broken off and chopped	4
6	pitted prunes, chopped	6
2 tbsp	chopped fresh parsley (or 1 tsp/5 mL dried)	30 mL
1	garlic clove, chopped	1

1. Place all ingredients in saucepan, bring to a boil, cover, and simmer for 30 to 40 minutes or until soft.
2. Add a bit of extra water at the end if you want it to be mushier, and let it be absorbed. Mash or purée to desired consistency. Makes about 4 cups (1 L).

NUTRITIONAL INFORMATION
A good source of protein, calcium, phosphorus, iron, and vitamins B and E.

STEAMED VEGETABLE FINGER FOODS

Steamed vegetables make healthy and tasty finger foods for your baby. Remember, this is a learning experience and a way for baby to practise his pincer grip, so expect a lot to land everywhere but in his mouth!

Your choice of
> Broccoli (peel stem to remove outer fibrous layer; use stem and florets)
>
> Carrots
>
> Cauliflower (remove stem)
>
> Beets
>
> Green beans
>
> Asparagus (trim about ½ inch/1 cm off bottom)

1. Peel or scrub vegetables and chop into small pieces that are easy to pick up with little fingers.
2. Steam until tender. Freeze in cube trays or on baking tray, then transfer to freezer storage bag.
3. Defrost in fridge overnight or drop a handful into boiled water, drain and serve.

SUPER-CHUNKY FOODS: 10 MONTHS+

The following recipes are suitable for babies ready for adult-like texture and can be offered well into toddlerhood as a main dish or accompaniment.

DELICIOUS LENTIL DAHL

Many people are surprised that their babies can eat spices like turmeric and cumin, but these add wonderful flavours, and turmeric is anti-inflammatory. Parents can eat this served over brown rice with a dollop of yogurt.

3 cups	water or no-sodium vegetable stock	750 mL
1 cup	red lentils, rinsed well	250 mL
1	medium sweet potato, chopped into small cubes	1
1	small onion, finely chopped	1
1 tbsp	extra-virgin olive oil	30 mL
1 tsp	turmeric	5 mL
1 tsp	cumin	5 mL
1	clove garlic, finely chopped	1
Handful	cilantro leaves	Handful
1 cup	packed baby spinach, finely chopped	250 mL
2	Swiss chard leaves, finely chopped	2
1	can (14 oz/398 mL) chickpeas, drained and rinsed	1

1. Combine water, lentils, sweet potato, onion, olive oil, turmeric, cumin, garlic, and cilantro in a medium saucepan. Bring to a boil, cover, and reduce heat. Simmer for about 20 minutes.
2. Add spinach and chard; simmer for 2 minutes. Stir in chickpeas and simmer for 3 minutes. Leave chunky or purée slightly to desired consistency.

NUTRITIONAL INFORMATION
A good source of vitamin C, vitamin A, magnesium, calcium, potassium, protein, and fibre.

Bean and Rice Surprise Stew

This is a more challenging texture, perfect for self-feeding and great for the whole family. The combination of beans and rice makes this purée a complete protein.

2 cups	water	500 mL
½ cup	brown rice, rinsed	125 mL
½ cup	chickpeas or adzuki beans, rinsed	125 mL
1	medium carrot, peeled and chopped	1
1	stalk celery, chopped	1
1 to 2	kale leaves, stems removed, finely chopped	1 to 2
1	small onion, finely chopped	1
1	clove garlic, minced	1
1	medium sweet potato, peeled and chopped	1
1 tbsp	fresh parsley	15 mL

1. Combine all ingredients in a medium saucepan and bring to a boil. Cover and simmer until rice is cooked and vegetables are tender, about 25 to 30 minutes. Makes about 3 cups (750 mL).

NUTRITIONAL INFORMATION
This purée is high in fibre, protein, manganese, potassium, iron, B vitamins, vitamin A, and vitamin C.

Fabulous Fruit

This fresh, raw purée is super yummy and is sure to please. Mom can make a little extra for herself and add some milk and protein powder for a healthy breakfast or snack. This is also a great purée to sneak some raw garlic into, if baby is getting sick.

2/3 cup	frozen wild blueberries	150 mL
1	avocado	1
1	ripe pear, cored	1
1	large banana	1

1. Purée all with a hand blender or mini food processor.
2. To increase the texture, purée ½ cup of the blueberries and simply stir in the rest of the fruit. Best made in small batches and eaten within two days. Can be frozen.

NUTRITIONAL INFORMATION
A good source of fibre, vitamin C, potassium, folic acid, and vitamin E.

Finger Food Pancakes

This is a great recipe the whole family can enjoy either as finger food or dipped in Yummy Carrot Spread or Delicious Lentil Dahl. Older ones will love this as breakfast drizzled with agave or maple syrup.

1 cup	brown rice flour	250 mL
¼ cup	potato starch	50 mL
¼ cup	tapioca starch	50 mL
2 tsp	baking powder	10 mL
1 tbsp	chia powder (Salba)	15 mL
1	egg yolk*	1
1 cup	(approx.) vanilla rice milk or unsweetened almond milk	250 mL
2 ½ tbsp	agave syrup	37 mL
3 tbsp	sunflower oil	45 mL

1. In a medium-sized bowl, whisk together brown rice flour, potato starch, tapioca starch, baking powder, and chia powder.
2. In a small bowl, whisk together the egg yolk, milk, and agave; slowly whisk in the oil. Pour over dry ingredients and mix thoroughly.
3. Heat a frying pan or griddle over medium-high heat and lightly coat with oil or butter. Pour 1 tablespoon (15 mL) batter per pancake into the frying pan. Cook each side until golden brown. Makes about 24 mini pancakes. Great for freezing!

* For eggless or vegan option, replace the egg with 3 tbsp/45 mL water mixed with 1 tbsp/15 mL ground flax. Let sit for a few minutes and add to wet ingredients. (*Note:* The vegan option produces a gummier texture.) You can also use whole egg once your baby turns one year old.

Option: Sprinkle cinnamon in the batter and serve with fruit purée. I also like to add grated carrot to the batter for some extra vegetable power.

NUTRITIONAL INFORMATION
Chia powder is one of nature's superfoods. It's a complex protein offering all eight amino acids, and it's high in fibre, omega-3 and omega-6, calcium, iron, folate, potassium, magnesium, and antioxidants. Agave syrup is a natural sweetener with trace amounts of calcium, potassium, magnesium, and iron. It has a low glycemic index, meaning that it doesn't affect blood sugar and insulin levels as sugar does.

BROWN RICE PUDDING

Serve as a meal or as a dessert.

1 ½ cups	water	375 mL
³/₄ cup	sweet brown rice, rinsed	175 mL
1	can (14 oz/398 mL) coconut milk	1
³/₄ cup	vanilla rice milk	175 mL
6	dried, unsulphured apricots, chopped	6
2 tbsp	chopped raisins	30 mL
1 tsp	cinnamon	5 mL
1	³/₄ inch (2 cm) piece ginger root, peeled	1

1. In a medium saucepan, bring water and sweet brown rice to a boil. Cover and simmer until all the water is absorbed and rice is nearly cooked.
2. Add coconut milk, vanilla rice milk, apricots, raisins, cinnamon, and ginger root and bring to a boil. Reduce heat and simmer, stirring often, until mixture thickens and rice is tender, about 10 to 15 minutes.
3. Remove ginger root and serve or freeze. Makes about 3 cups (750 mL).

Note: You can also use short grain brown rice.

NUTRITIONAL INFORMATION
Brown rice is a whole grain providing a great source of fibre, manganese, selenium, magnesium, and B vitamins.

FRUITY CURRY BUCKWHEAT

Don't let the curry put you off from making this for your baby—it's deliciously sweet, and babies love it! Containing buckwheat, this gluten-free purée is easy to digest and is a very good source of protein, B vitamins, iron, and calcium. Use buckwheat groats, not toasted buckwheat or kashi.

2 to 2 ½ cups	water	500–750 mL
3	nectarines or 1 large mango, finely chopped	3
⅓ cup	raisins	75 mL
½	onion, finely chopped	½
1	clove garlic, finely chopped	1
1 to 2 tsp	curry powder	5–10 mL
1 to 2 tsp	cinnamon	5–10 mL
1 cup	buckwheat groats, rinsed quickly	250 mL
2	curly kale leaves, stems removed and finely chopped	2

1. In a medium saucepan, combine the water, nectarines or mango, raisins, onion, garlic, curry powder, and cinnamon. Bring to a boil, then stir in buckwheat and kale.
2. Simmer for about 10 minutes or until the buckwheat is soft, stirring frequently. The mixture can be left chunky, or puréed for a smoother texture. Makes about 3 cups (750 mL).

NUTRITIONAL INFORMATION
Buckwheat is a gluten-free grain from the rhubarb family. It contains protein and B vitamins and is rich in phosphorus, potassium, iron, and calcium.

Baby's First Chicken or Turkey

Although I recommend offering meat closer to one year of age, some parents prefer to introduce it earlier. Here's a great recipe that offers lots of fibre as well as protein, but make sure that you use dark meat as it's higher in iron. Offer two to three times a week only, not every day.

1 tbsp	extra-virgin olive oil	15 mL
1	small onion, chopped	1
½ cup	(approx.) organic chicken or turkey (dark meat), cut into chunks	125 g
1	medium carrot, peeled and chopped into small cubes	1
1 ¼ cups	sweet potato, peeled and chopped	300 mL
1 ¼ cups	water or no-sodium chicken stock	300 mL

1. Heat the oil in a medium saucepan and add the onion. Sauté for 3 to 5 minutes or until soft. Add the chicken or turkey and sauté 3 to 5 minutes longer. Stir in carrot, sweet potato, and water or stock, and bring to a boil.

2. Simmer, covered, for about 30 minutes or until chicken is cooked through and vegetables are tender. Purée to desired consistency. Makes about 3 cups (750 mL).

NUTRITIONAL INFORMATION
A good source of protein, fibre, niacin, phosphorus, calcium, iron, zinc, and vitamins B6, B12, C, and D.

BABY'S FIRST FISH

As mentioned above, I suggest introducing meat protein slowly. Fish is a potential allergen, so go slow with this one. For a tasty dish the whole family will enjoy, serve some before puréeing.

1 tbsp	extra-virgin olive oil	15 mL
1	medium onion, chopped	1
2 ½ cups	water	625 mL
1 cup	brown rice, rinsed	250 mL
½ pound	(approx.) cod, skinned and filleted, cut into cubes*	250 g
3/4 cup	peas	200 mL
1	carrot, peeled and chopped	1
1/4 cup	fresh parsley or cilantro, chopped	50 mL
1	clove garlic, minced	1

1. Heat the oil in a medium saucepan. Add the onion and cook until tender, about 3 to 5 minutes. Stir in water, rice, cod, peas, carrot, parsley, and garlic. Simmer for about 30 minutes or until the rice is tender.
2. Purée until you reach the desired texture. Makes about 3 cups (750 mL).

* Haddock or sole can be substituted.

NUTRITIONAL INFORMATION
A good source of protein, fibre, selenium, manganese, magnesium, B vitamins, omega-3 fatty acids, and vitamin D.

Yummy Carrot Spread

A very versatile spread that can be eaten straight up, or spread over Finger Food Pancakes or rice cakes. For toddlers, serve it as a dip with raw veggies and crackers. This also makes a great sandwich spread.

8	medium carrots, peeled and diced	8
1	clove garlic	1
1 tbsp	tahini or sunflower seed butter	15 mL
1 tbsp	fresh cilantro or basil, chopped	15 mL
1 tbsp	extra-virgin olive or flax oil	15 mL
1 tsp	lemon juice	5 mL

1. Steam carrots until tender and cool slightly.
2. In a small bowl, combine carrots with garlic, tahini, cilantro, olive oil, and lemon juice. Purée with a hand blender. Makes about 1 ½ cups (375 mL). Best consumed within three days, this purée also can be frozen, although the texture might change slightly.

NUTRITIONAL INFORMATION
Carrots are an excellent source of antioxidant compounds and the richest vegetable source of the pro-vitamin A carotenes.

BEANY GREEN DIP

Bursting with fresh flavour!

1	can (14 oz/398 mL) cannellini beans	1
1	garlic clove, roughly chopped	1
1/3 cup	basil or cilantro, roughly chopped	75 mL
1/4 cup	extra-virgin or flax oil	50 mL
4 tsp	(approx.) lemon juice	20 mL
1/4 tsp	paprika	1 mL
1/4 tsp	cumin	1 mL
Handful	dinosaur kale, chopped (optional)	Handful

1. Purée all ingredients in a food processor or with a hand blender—then it's ready to eat! Makes about 1 ½ cups (375 mL). It's best eaten fresh but can be frozen.

NUTRITIONAL INFORMATION
A good source of fibre, protein, iron, magnesium, folate, vitamin A, and calcium.

SPICED-UP APPLES

This is a great purée to add to plain organic yogurt if you're feeding your baby dairy. For a subtle twist, try making this recipe with half apples and half pears.

8	medium apples (Gala, Fuji, or Pink Lady)	8
½ tsp	ground cinnamon	2 mL
¼ tsp	grated lemon zest or juice	1 mL
Pinch	ground ginger	Pinch
Pinch	ground nutmeg (optional)	Pinch

1. Peel, core, and chop apples into small cubes.
2. Steam apples until tender. Transfer to a bowl and stir in cinnamon, lemon zest, and ginger. Purée to desired consistency. Makes about 2 cups (500 mL).

NUTRITIONAL INFORMATION
A good source of fibre, vitamin C, and flavonoids.

Hummus

Hummus is fantastic served on its own or spread on a rice cake. Instead of raw garlic, you can use roasted garlic for a sweeter, milder flavour. Remember that you're not adding salt, so don't expect this to taste like store-bought.

1	can (14 oz/398 mL) chickpeas, rinsed	1	
4 tbsp	(approx.) extra-virgin olive oil	60 mL	
2 tbsp	(approx.) water	30 mL	
2 tbsp	tahini (sesame seed paste)	30 mL	
2 tbsp	lemon juice	30 mL	
1	clove garlic	1	

1. Place all ingredients in a bowl or food processor and blend to desired consistency, adding extra water to thin it out or extra olive oil for more flavour. Makes about 2 cups (500 mL).

To make roasted garlic: Slice the top off a whole garlic bulb and place in aluminum foil. Drizzle with extra-virgin olive oil, wrap the foil together, and bake in a 350°F (180°C) oven for about 20 minutes or until cloves are tender. Cool, and "squish" garlic cloves out of the bulb.

NUTRITIONAL INFORMATION
A good source of fibre, calcium, magnesium, iron, folate, manganese, copper, and protein.

BABY'S FIRST BIRTHDAY CAKE

I'm always being asked for a healthy birthday cake recipe for those wanting to offer cake to baby too. Offering a sugary wheat cake with food-coloured icing may cause symptoms in your baby if she hasn't eaten it before, so here's a recipe she'll love. You can also bake the batter in mini muffin tins for cupcakes that are the perfect size for little hands! You can make this recipe with spelt or wheat flour—simply omit the xanthan gum.

4 cups	all-purpose gluten-free flour mix* (such as Bob's Red Mill)	1 L
2 tbsp	baking powder	30 mL
2 tsp	xanthan gum	10 mL
1 tsp	cinnamon	5 mL
½ tsp	sea salt	2 mL
½ tsp	cardamom (optional)	2 mL
¼ tsp	nutmeg	1 mL
1 cup	vanilla rice milk	250 mL
1 cup	apple or pear juice	250 mL
½ cup	sunflower oil	125 mL
½ cup	maple syrup	125 mL
1 tbsp	vanilla	15 mL
2 cups	grated carrots	500 mL
½ cup	raisins (soaked in hot water and drained)	125 mL
½ cup	walnuts or sunflower seeds, chopped	125 mL

1. In a large mixing bowl, combine the flour, baking powder, xanthan gum, cinnamon, salt, cardamom, and nutmeg.

2. In a medium-sized bowl, combine the rice milk, apple juice, sunflower oil, maple syrup, and vanilla. Stir in the grated carrots. Add to the dry ingredients and blend thoroughly in a mixer with the paddle attachment. Add raisins and walnuts and mix thoroughly.

3. Pour batter into two lightly greased 9-inch (1.5 L) round baking pans. Bake in 350°F (180°C) oven for about 30 to 35 minutes, or until a toothpick inserted in

the centre comes out dry. Cool on rack before frosting with Sweet Potato Icing. Makes 1 double-layer cake.

* Or make your own gluten-free flour mix of 3 cups brown rice flour, ½ cup potato starch, and ½ cup tapioca starch.

Sweet Potato Icing

4	medium sweet potatoes	4
½ tsp	cinnamon	2 mL
2 tbsp	maple or agave syrup	30 mL

1. Bake the sweet potatoes in a 350°F (180°C) oven for 15 to 20 minutes, or until soft. Score the skin and squeeze the sweet potato out into a food processor or bowl. Add cinnamon and syrup and process or beat until smooth. Adjust to taste and refrigerate until ready to use. Makes approximately 1 ½ cups (375 mL).

NUTRITIONAL INFORMATION
This is a sugar-free, gluten-free, and dairy-free cake that everyone will enjoy. Carrots are high in beta carotene, and walnuts and sunflower seeds are high in omega-3 and -6 essential fats, calcium, magnesium, and trace minerals.

THE NEXT STAGE: 9- TO 12-MONTH FEEDING CHART

The following table is to be used as a guideline for the milk/solid schedule for 9- to 12-month-olds.

Start to offer water in a sippy cup throughout the day.

This table shows you how to introduce and test new textured purées for five days, in this case, lentil purée. All other food eaten at other meals should already have been eaten and on the safe list.

	Upon Rising	Breakfast	Sleep	Lunch	Sleep	Dinner	Bedtime
Day 1	Milk*	Avocado and Pear, Blueberry, or Banana Purée	Milk	Milk + Introduction to Lentils	Milk	Milk + Zucchini Purée mixed with amaranth or millet puffs	Milk
Day 2	Milk	Pea and Mint Purée	Milk	Milk + Broccoli Purée mixed with quinoa puffs	Milk	Milk + Introduction to Lentils	Milk
Day 3	Milk	Sweet Potato Purée with cinnamon	Milk	Introduction to Lentils	Milk	Broccoli or Green Bean Purée and Apricot Purée	Milk
Day 4	Milk	Introduction to Lentils	Milk	Milk + Green Bean Purée	Milk	Avocado and Pear Purée	Milk
Day 5	Milk	Oat Cereal mixed with Spiced-Up Apples	Milk	Introduction to Lentils	Milk	Butternut Squash and Parsnip Purée	Milk

* Milk is either breast milk or formula.

TODDLER TIMES
12 Months and Beyond

Toddlerhood was one of my favourite stages as I started to see my baby growing into a little person. She was becoming more independent and was remarkably clever at figuring out how certain toys or games worked (or she tried, anyway); she also knew what she wanted, and it took some inventive distracting to sway her! She started cruising along the couch and would take the odd step when she wasn't thinking about it, and she insisted on practising other new skills all the time. Mealtimes took on a whole new dynamic, as she began self-feeding and asserting her preferences. Although she couldn't talk back to me just yet, we could still have a conversation about all sorts of things, including food and what we were eating.

WHAT'S YOUR TODDLER EATING NOW?

Your baby has probably had a great appetite up until now (other than when sick or teething), but you might see that slow down. His weight plateaus as he becomes a busybody and gets into everything except what might be on his plate. Grazing or snacking becomes more important now as his milk intake declines, making way for more nutrients and calories from food.

Ideally, mealtimes continue to be lots of fun, with a wide variety of tastes and textures on the menu. But perhaps your toddler has limited tastes for certain foods. I encourage you to keep trying with foods that he isn't sure about or dislikes. What he will eat in terms of flavours and textures can change daily, and if it's not on the menu, you won't know if it could be his next favourite food.

By around one year, your toddler may be eating a long list of foods, including lots of colourful fruits and vegetables, some grains and breads, beans, pulses (lentils) and legumes, and maybe dairy, eggs, meat, and fish. If any of these haven't been offered yet, you can start to introduce them any time now. Egg whites and honey are now on the OK list, so try scrambled eggs, French toast, or omelettes. Texture is often a hurdle that your toddler will need some time to get over. Meat, for instance, may not be eaten on its own until 18 months, or fish might need to be surrounded by potato in a fish cake or fish bake.

Keep experimenting with an array of colourful vegetables mixed with beans and rice or with something new like buckwheat (see Fruity Curry Buckwheat on page 213), which may have had too much texture when you tried it last; try it again and see what happens! Your toddler may now gobble up cooked quinoa with veg-etables before it's puréed (see Introducing Quinoa page 205), or it could still have too much texture. You can only move at your child's speed—although your friend's toddler may be eating anything and everything, don't think that he should be doing the same. We all have different preferences for textures and flavours, and this also applies to your toddler.

RAISING A VEGETARIAN OR VEGAN TODDLER

I have counselled many parents who prefer their children to be raised with the same dietary philosophy as the rest of the family. Eating a vegetarian diet can be healthy, as long as you know how to create a meal with complex protein and ensure the common nutrient deficiencies (iron, zinc, B12, omega-3 essential fats, including DHA) are covered. In my practice, I recommend that babies eat a predominantly vegetarian diet until about age one—these babies grow into strong and healthy toddlers. At about nine months, I suggest giving organic egg yolk (if baby's not allergic), which provides complex animal protein and miner-als that are important for growth—and can be a great fit for a vegetarian diet. If you're raising your child on a vegan diet, supplement with DHA from an algae source as well as with vitamin B12, and learn which foods supply iron and zinc (see the list of vitamins and minerals from food in the Resources). It's easy for your little one to become deficient in these nutrients, and with such a huge growth rate between 18 months and three years, she needs nutritional support to reach her full potential.

Vegetarians often lack protein in their diet, but offering protein-rich eggs and fish, if you're able to, can cover this concern. Protein provides the building blocks (amino acid) for cell growth and repair, supports a strong and healthy immune system, and stabilizes blood sugar. Animal protein offers minerals such as iron, zinc, and vitamin B12 in more absorbable forms than vegetarian protein, but you can make up for this difference by eating smart. Serving foods high in vitamin C alongside iron-rich beans, lentils, quinoa, amaranth, soy, blackstrap molasses, and sunflower, pumpkin, and sesame seeds increases iron absorption. Moving to a full vegetarian diet at school age or adolescence may be a better nutritional choice; however, your toddler may have decided that meat isn't on his menu just yet.

To ensure adequate calorie intake from a vegetarian diet, some higher-fat foods need to be eaten. Nut and seeds, coconut milk or oil, eggs, and dairy products are all great choices. Your toddler is busy and needs a constant supply of calories. Fats provide higher calories, at nine calories per gram of fat, than protein or carbohydrate, at four calories per gram. While carbohydrates are also important, these are easy foods to get into the diet (fruits, vegetables, cereals, and grains). I rarely see children who suffer from a lack of carbohydrates. Make sure that protein, fat, and carbohydrate are offered to your toddler every day.

What You Need to Know about Soy

Soy products are not always the best protein option for vegetarian diets. Items such as tofu, tempeh, milk, edamame, oil, or sauce have the potential to be allergenic, and they also contain a compound called phytate. Phytate binds with minerals such as iron, zinc, and calcium and interferes with their absorption by the body, which isn't ideal for supporting strong bone growth, especially for vegetarians trying to eat iron- and zinc-rich foods. Furthermore, almost all nonorganic soy is genetically modified, which, as we saw in Chapter 5, may bring negative health issues in the future.

IT'S OK TO PURÉE

As your baby reaches age one, you may expect that her eating will change dramatically and she'll start eating family meals or food from your plate. But please don't worry if she still wants her purée or prefers her own food. Purée can be made with so many great foods, nutrients, herbs, and spices that you otherwise wouldn't be able to get your toddler to eat, so I'd encourage serving it for as long as you can. Leafy greens, which are packed with nutrients, are difficult to give without puréeing because they're a choking hazard. Try adding spinach, chard, kale, parsley, cilantro, or maybe a vegetable that's not a favourite, such as broccoli or cauliflower, to a purée. The purées will eventually get chunkier and lumpier, and before you know it (usually around 18 months to two years), your toddler will have transitioned to table food and you'll be cooking one meal for the whole family. Now all you have to do is make healthy family meals!

TIME FOR THE SWITCH TO MILK

> ### From the Mouths of Moms: My Signing Story
>
> My husband and I learned baby sign language when our first daughter was about 9 months old. She showed us her first sign at 11 months by signing *fan* as she looked at a ceiling fan. As she got older, we kept showing her the signs for *more, finished, hungry, drink, milk,* and the different names of foods. It was slow to start, but she ended up becoming a signing machine and communicating to us what she wanted, when she was hungry, and if she wanted something specifically, such as an apple or a pear. Signing really helped reduce her frustration with not being understood and was incredibly helpful at mealtimes. It also allowed us to teach her the names of as many fruits and vegetables we could find signs for. Crackers were a firm favourite, so that was a sign she learned quickly!

At about one year, formula-fed babies will transition from formula to milk, which will provide needed calories and nutrients throughout the day. Formula is needed up until one year because it makes up baby's main source of nutrition. If your one-year-old is still on a limited diet or not a great eater, you can choose to keep him on formula until 13 or 14 months or until the diet expands and he eats more.

If breastfeeding, you can continue nursing morning and night or more often if you're home with your toddler. Or you might choose to wean completely from the breast at this point, whether you're heading back to work or not. I encourage you to keep breastfeeding for as long as possible.

Either way, you can introduce a drink of milk from age one. A bottle or nurse first thing in the morning and before bed is recommended until close to two years. Between 12 and 18 months, your baby's milk intake should start to decrease as her food intake increases. Ideally, your toddler will be eating three meals a day plus snacks and working toward decreasing her milk to about 16 oz (473 mL) per day, or maybe less.

If your toddler is drinking three or four bottles of formula or milk a day, start to decrease the amount you offer. With a full belly of milk, he isn't going to be as hungry for a plate of fruits, vegetables, carbohydrates, and protein-rich foods, and you might think he's being a picky eater and just doesn't want to eat. Drinking too much milk also lowers the amount of nutrients that can be gained from other foods—milk offers a certain nutrient profile, but your toddler needs more than just calcium, vitamin D, and fat from milk in his diet.

MILK OPTIONS

I know you're thinking options ... what options? Well, not everyone does well with dairy or cow's milk, so you might need to choose another kind. I've mentioned before that milk is the most allergenic food. Whether you can't offer it because of a reaction to dairy in the past or don't want to offer your toddler as much as she might choose to drink, milk is still necessary to keep up with her calorie needs. Higher-fat milks are recommended for all toddlers. Your options are:

- homogenized (3.38%) cow's milk, preferably organic;
- goat's milk (3.25%), preferably organic;
- sheep's milk (6%); and
- almond milk, preferably organic and homemade.

Cow's Milk

If tolerated, cow's milk is a good source of calcium, vitamin D, and protein. Look out for possible signs of sensitivity such as diarrhea, rash (including eczema), runny nose, or constant cold. These symptoms may occur with increasing amounts of milk. An allergy to milk will show more severe reactions, including hives, vomiting, blood in the stool, and swelling.

Goat's Milk

Goat's milk is a great alternative to cow's milk and offers similar nutritional benefits. Children intolerant to cow's milk are often able to consume goat's milk without any symptoms. A goat is a smaller animal, so its milk is easier for humans to digest than cow's milk. It's naturally homogenized, which may make the fat easier to digest. Also, goat's milk proteins have a slightly different amino acid structure, so an allergy is less likely. Goat's milk is a very good source of calcium, protein, phosphorus, potassium, vitamin B2, and the amino acid tryptophan. A common concern with drinking goat's milk is that it's low in folic acid. Check the packaging to see that it's fortified with folic acid (most brands are).

Sheep's Milk

Sheep's milk is more nutritious and better tolerated than cow's or goat's milk. Many common symptoms of diarrhea, nausea, vomiting, rash, migraine, and congestion disappear when drinking sheep's milk. It's high in protein, and rich in calcium, magnesium, phosphorus, potassium, zinc, vitamins A, C, and D, folate, and B12. Although it has a high fat content, 25 percent is medium chain triglycerides—healthy fats that are easily digested, not stored in the body as fat, and also help to reduce cholesterol. Sheep's milk may not be as easy to find as goat's milk, but if your local health food store sells sheep's milk products, such as cheese or yogurt, they might be able to order it for you.

The following table compares the nutrients in cow's, goat's, and sheep's milk.

NUTRIENT COMPARISON OF COW'S, GOAT'S, AND SHEEP'S MILK

Nutrients	Cow's Milk (3.3%)	Goat's Milk (3.25%)	Sheep's Milk (6%)
Serving	250 mL	250 mL	250 mL
Energy	155 cal	167 cal	256 cal
Protein	8 g	9 g	15 g
Carbohydrates	12 g	11 g	13 g
Fat	8 g	10 g	17 g
Saturated fat	5.4 g	6.5 g	11 g
Calcium	291 mg	326 mg	483 mg
Iron	0.1 mg	0.12 mg	0.15 mg
Sodium	103 mg	122 mg	108 mg
Potassium	369 mg	499 mg	365 mg
Magnesium	26 mg	34 mg	75 mg
Phosphorus	235 mg	270 mg	332 mg
Vitamin A	72 RAE	136.64 RAE	360 iu
Vitamin D	2.7 mcg	0.73 mcg	2.2 mcg
Folate	13 DFE	2.4 mcg	1.35 mcg
B12	1.13 mcg	0.16 mcg	0.711 mg
Riboflavin (B2)	0.47 mg	0.34 mg	1 mg

Mcg: microgram (sometimes seen as µg).

iu: international unit

RAE: Vitamin A and carotenoids are measured differently. Animal foods contain vitamin A, and vegetables and legumes, beta carotene (carotenoids). Using the measurement RAE helps to account for those differences. Here is the formula: 1 ug vitamin A = 12 ug carotenoids = 1 RAE.

DFE: Dietary Folate Equivalents—used because of the different bioavailability of folates and folic acid. 1µg DFE= 1 µg of food folate = 0.5 µg of folic acid taken on an empty stomach = 0.6 µg of folic acid from fortified food or as a supplement taken with meals.

Almond Milk

Almonds are a powerhouse of nutrients, including heart-healthy monounsaturated fats, which are associated with a reduced risk of heart disease. Almonds are a very good source of vitamin E, omega-6 fatty acids, calcium, phosphorus, manganese, magnesium, copper, and vitamin B2.

I recommend making your own almond milk or looking for unsweetened options, as commercial milks can be high in sugar and additives, as well as not providing nearly the same benefits as whole almonds. If you look at the label of most ready-to-drink almond milks, they're made with blanched almonds (without the nutritious skins) and contain high levels of sugar.

If you're feeding your toddler almond milk, you'll need to add four table-spoons (60 mL) of full-fat coconut milk to four cups (1 L) of almond milk to increase the amount of saturated fat and calories so the nutritional profile is more like that of cow's or goat's milk.

Rice milk alone is not suitable for a toddler as a replacement for cow's milk. It's fortified with calcium but lacks the fat needed for extra calories. Rice milk could be mixed with almond or cow's milk from about 18 months of age as long as the overall diet contains extra fat to make up for getting less from the milk.

I've seen many toddlers who choose not to drink milk. It doesn't matter what vessel it comes in—bottle, sippy cup, or glass with a straw—they just don't take to it. If this is the case with your toddler, please don't be concerned. Look at the rest of his dairy intake from, say, yogurt, cheese, or cottage cheese—if any of those foods are a part of his diet, he's covered. Although milk is an important drink for the calories it provides, these can easily be made up with foods instead.

HEALTHY TODDLER SNACKS

Snacking is incredibly important for your toddler. Her breast milk or formula might have been her main snack (and might still be), but now it's time to offer food as snacks and reduce the amount of milk (if she's still drinking more than 16 to 24 oz/473 to 710 mL). Her busy body needs a constant source of nourishment and calories. Her little stomach can't hold enough food to keep her going from breakfast 'til lunch or lunch 'til dinner, especially when her intake at meal-time might sometimes be hit-and-miss.

Getting the quantity of snacks right so that mealtime isn't affected is some-times a challenge, but keeping to a routine of snack and mealtime helps toddlers' bodies tremendously to maintain a good blood sugar balance.

Snack trays with flip lids are a great invention. In our house it was as much fun to flip the lids open and shut as it was to find out what was in each compart-ment. And then there was the fun of discovering the character at the bottom of the tray once the food was all gone. It all helps create healthy associations with food.

Snacks of fruit and vegetables cut into pieces that aren't easily choked on are preferable to cookies, chips, or sweet treats. Hummus, baba ganoush, or my Beany Green Dip (see page 217) are often good fun and can be packed with nutrients. Whether your toddler eats it straight up or as a dip with the cracker or carrot stick acting as a spoon, if it goes down the hatch, it's all good!

Some healthy snack suggestions include:

- Fresh or frozen wild blueberries. Frozen are better eaten seated at a table, as they can be pretty messy.
- Cut-up organic grapes (conventional grapes are heavily sprayed with pesticides).
- Banana slices (cut in half or quartered), plain or with a dollop of almond butter or tahini on top.
- Plain yogurt mixed with fruit purée or frozen blueberries.
- Rice cakes or crackers with hummus, baba ganoush, Yummy Carrot Spread*, or almond butter topped with apple butter or fruit spread (jam sweetened with juice).
- Dried fruit such as raisins, apples, apricots, or "fruit leather" strips with cow's, goat's, or sheep's milk cheese.
- Smoothies made with banana, blueberry, pear, or mango and blended with an alternative milk (rice or almond) and some hemp protein powder.*
- Flake cereal, Barbara's Breakfast O's, and/or rice puffs.
- Organic Rice Crisp Surprise Squares.*
- Go Faster Granola Bars.*
- Sneaky Little Muffins.*
- No-Mess Fruity Pops.*
- Fruity Frozen Yogurt.*
- Steamed veggie sticks: carrot, parsnip, beets, or even broccoli.

* See the end of the chapter for recipes.

SNACKS AND BABY'S TEETH

I interviewed three dentists for their views on childhood cavities and how they seem to be increasing, and they all agreed that snacking or grazing all day is not good for oral health. They commented that dried fruits are healthy but sticky and can hang around on the bite surface of premolars or molars or get stuck in between teeth. All three preferred that snacks be eaten at one sitting. Grazing changes the pH of the mouth to acid, whereas an alkaline environment protects teeth from bacteria and therefore cavities. Eating a piece of cheese or a carrot stick at the end of a snack helps to alkalize the mouth after eating raisins, for instance. Dr. Dana Colson explains, "The mouth doesn't recognize the difference between all the different sugars; honey, refined sugar, sugary drinks, candy, and raisins—it can all have the same end result. Plaque takes the sugar and turns it to acid and then causes destruction of enamel." Brushing or even wiping the teeth after sticky snacks is essential to fight off cavities.

UPSIDE-DOWN BOWL NIGHT

In our house, we've always encouraged food that's "good for your body" and helps you grow big and strong, run faster, and play longer. We've used simple language to plant the seeds in their minds that will grow into an awareness of what's healthy to eat and what needs to be eaten in moderation. So far, we have very healthy children who have a great approach to a nutritious eating.

It's not just organic kale and broccoli around our house, though, and sometimes it can take a bit of coaxing to get the girls to eat what we would like them to. My husband gets involved in this process. He chops apples into moon and star shapes and cucumber into butterflies, and he also invented what is now a famous tradition (with our friends, anyway): Upside-Down Bowl Night. As soon as it's mentioned, all the food on the girls' dinner plates is gobbled up! Start with a plate with something really good on it, such as pure fruit sorbet or Divine Cookies (see the recipe on page 262). Next, take a cereal-sized bowl and turn it upside down over the yummy stuff. Put something that you want your toddler to eat—fruit or something you're seeing resistance to (we've used broccoli)—on top of the bottom of the bowl. She has to eat what's on top of her bowl before she can reveal what's underneath, and it should be worth the wait. Everyone at the table has to turn their bowl right side up at the same time. Genius! Try it out as your toddler gets older and can understand what's happening. We save this as a treat for week-ends or when friends come over now, as the girls wanted it every night.

ANY FOODS STILL TO AVOID?

Some doctors recommend continuing to avoid peanuts until closer to age three. However, if you don't have any allergies in the family or siblings with eczema or asthma, and the introduction of solids up to now has been smooth sailing, then you might do a controlled introduction by placing a small amount on the inside of your toddler's lip. Don't offer anything new for a few days. You can do the same with almonds and sesame if you haven't tried them yet (be aware that hummus has tahini in it). Look out for hives, rash, swelling, or eczema getting worse. Other highly allergenic foods include seafood and fish, although fish is slightly less so than seafood. Try them when you feel confident that you're in the clear for allergic symptoms.

Food intolerance can happen at any time, as it's more common when intake of a specific food increases. Wheat and dairy are both common food sensitivities, along with corn, soy, sugar, chocolate, and sometimes the gluten-containing grains (rye, barley, kamut, spelt, and, some say, oats). As dairy increases in the diet from yogurt, cheese, and milk, your child might show symptoms of a con-stant runny nose because dairy products are mucus-forming. Although it typi-cally leads to gassiness and constipation, wheat also may cause the constant runny nose. Every now and then, keep a food diary and see which symptoms might correlate with foods that are eaten every day or at more than one meal a day. Wheat, dairy, and corn are foods that are often hiding in prepackaged foods, from cookies to ice cream and "healthy" snack bars. See Chapter 7 for more on allergy and intolerance.

Avoid sugar as much as possible. Your toddler doesn't need it in the amount that's found in so many foods. Read labels and look out for cane juice or syrup, or any other description of cane sugar. It's still sugar, though it's not always pre-sented as such. Look at the ingredient list, not just the nutritional composition. Carbohydrate foods, such as rice cakes, will show as "sugar" in the nutritional composition chart, although they might not contain refined sugar. Sugar is found in just about every food that you don't make yourself and can encourage a sweet tooth in your toddler, leading him to refuse more nutritious foods for a healthy body. I have even seen cane syrup in gummy vitamins for children—that's a combination most dentists would love to ban. Along with causing cavities, sugar slows down the immune's response to foreign invaders, can trigger behavioural problems, and may create blood sugar imbalances, and it will keep your toddler going for only short periods when what he needs is a continuous energy supply.

IMPORTANT NUTRIENTS FOR SUPER-HEALTHY TODDLERS

Essential nutrients in the toddler years are the B vitamins, essential fatty acids (omega-3 and omega-6), vitamin C, and zinc. B vitamins provide energy, vitamin C contributes to a strong immune system (as is zinc), and zinc is important for growth.

EFAs (especially DHA) support development of nerve cells in the spine and brain. As your toddler becomes more active and dexterous with her limbs, her nutrient intake needs to increase to support the nervous system's development, allowing for speed and agility of movement as well as sharp mental focus. Eighteen months of age to three years is one of the most rapid growth periods for the spinal column (other than in utero) as the muscular system around it develops to support the full range of flexibility. Studies show that higher levels of EFAs in the diet can increase IQ, mental focus, and concentration, and help reduce symptoms of hyperactivity.

Avoiding the Picky Eater

You may have experienced challenges with feeding your toddler, or you may be lucky and have a great eater. It's common for your toddler to show his likes, preferences, and dislikes and to change them weekly! Your job is to be creative and come up with new foods in different forms and continue to reinvent.

When to worry? If your toddler's eating only a few foods, suffering from recurrent colds and infections, has behavioural problems (possibly due to low blood sugar), and/or is losing weight, that's when it's time to seek help. Tissue salts, mineral salts that are very low dose but have high absorbability, can be used to increase nutrient status as well as mineral absorption from foods. Picky eating can often be a vicious cycle of not eating and then failing to get the essential nutrients that stimulate appetite. Be sure to rule out iron deficiency, which can lead to a lack of appetite.

Try to identify why your child refuses to eat. Refusing food may be an emotional plea for attention or a way of rebelling against change, such as mom going back to work. If a toddler doesn't want mom to leave, she might refuse breakfast knowing that she'll stay longer to feed her. It's her way of controlling the situation, especially when she sees a reaction. These issues may need to be addressed on a different level than just eating.

Make mealtimes relaxing and fun. Involve your toddler in meal preparation and cooking. Give foods names (such as "trees" for broccoli), or associate it with a favourite character. Maximize on textures he likes—the dry texture of bread, chewy noodles, or wet oatmeal. Sit with your toddler at each meal, eat with him, and encourage him when he eats something. If he's old enough, ask for a certain amount of bites before he leaves the table and have the fanfare ready when he achieves it. Don't make eating a struggle. That will kill his appetite, and the battle won't necessarily go the way you want it to.

"My toddler will only eat ..." I've heard it hundreds of times from parents. "My toddler will only eat cheese, bread, chicken pieces, or french fries." If it's not in the house or offered when you're out, then it can't be eaten. Simple. Your toddler might have a strong personality and insist on what he wants, but you're still in charge, so don't offer what you don't want him to eat. If you're out and about and are stuck for something to eat, don't venture into a fast-food restaurant with limited healthy choices—go down the road for falafel or sushi (vegetarian, as he might not be ready for raw fish), or just pick up some fruit or raisins to keep him going until you can find some healthy food. The only way that a toddler will start to eat unhealthy food is if you allow it.

To be sure that she isn't living on air (as it sometimes seems), look at what she has eaten in a whole day and week, rather than at just one meal. If she's at daycare or isn't with you during the day, when was her last snack? How much did she eat today, or what did she eat yesterday? If yesterday was a food-filled day, she might hardly touch her plate today. Again, a food diary with times of snacks or meals can really help to alleviate your stress and lessen mealtime pressure. Start talking about why she is eating, how the foods will help to make her strong and keep her healthy. Relate that to something that makes sense. "In order to play all day long at the park with your friends, you need to eat good food."

Here are some other healthy-eating ideas:

- Encourage snacking every couple of hours. If mealtimes aren't going well, offer snacks of pieces of chicken and peas, for instance. Toddlers need about 40 calories per inch of height per day. They burn calories quickly so need constant topping up.
- Have friends over to show them how it's done. Children are influenced by what others do even at a young age, so seeing their friends clean their plates might just inspire them to try too.
- Be inventive with the way you cut up food. Make special shapes and give them names.
- Sneak fruits or vegetables into everything! Chop or process them very small and add to Super Chicken Burgers (see page 258), under the cheese topping of pizza, and into bean dips, puréed soup, or pasta sauce. This way they can't easily identify or pick out what they don't want to eat.
- Serve their meals or snacks at their own table. A kid-sized table may be more appealing than the big table or high chair. Let them know that big girls and boys can sit at their own table, but only if they eat what's on their plates.
- Don't worry about which meal happens when. We are accustomed to eating breakfast-type foods in the morning, but it's not necessary to follow that schedule. Still aim for a variety of foods, not just cereal for breakfast, lunch, and dinner. If they're not eating much, make what does get eaten count.
- If your toddler is inconsistent with foods that you have lovingly prepared, don't take it personally, and don't stop offering the same or new foods.

OFF TO DAYCARE: AVOIDING SICKNESS AND DEALING WITH SOMEONE ELSE'S MENU

Daycare is one of the most dreaded situations of the parents I speak with. Being home for almost a year and watching your baby grow up into a little person is precious. And now it's time to drop him off at the door of a place you put your trust in and walk away, praying that it's all going to be OK. The transition can be heartwrenching at the beginning, but it quickly improves as your toddler realizes what fun daycare is.

When you're doing the rounds of daycares or making child care arrangements, ask to see a menu of the food served. If you aren't sure about some of the foods on the menu, ask if you can bring your own food. Most daycare centres don't permit nuts because they're a potential allergen. Ask if you can use sunflower, pumpkin, or sesame seed butters instead of peanut or almond butter. Look into how much of the food is organic, and how much wheat and dairy is served. In my consultations with daycares to improve their menus, I spend most of my time suggesting grain alternatives to wheat. Wheat is in just about everything and is offered three to four times a day in the form of bread, buns, cookies, crackers, cereal, and muffins. What do they give the children to drink? How easy would it be to give them water instead of juice, and do you want them having milk? All these questions need to be answered to help you decide which child care situation is best for your toddler. I've heard of parents turning down a daycare spot because hot dogs, chicken nuggets, and Jell-O were on the menu. I'm astounded that anyone would think that's an appropriate diet for a growing child.

Once you have the food situation figured out, it's time to boost everyone's immune system. It's common for everyone to come down with some sort of sickness during the first year of daycare. As I discussed in Chapter 7, your baby's immune system needs to be put through its paces, so the sneezes and wheezes that accompany children in daycare do serve a purpose! It's crazy how long a cold can last, or how you can be sick from September to March. I remember when my youngest was just over a year, she and I were both sick for a whole month (as well as off and on for most of the winter). Luckily, neither of us got a secondary infection (ear, chest, or throat infection) that required antibiotics. Our immune systems worked really hard to keep the illness under control with the support of loads of vitamin C, garlic, echinacea, and rest.

My definition of a strong immune system is one that's able to fight off illness and diseases that come your way through viruses, bacteria, fungi, or parasites. Colds and sickness will happen (especially during teething episodes, when the immune system is busy thinking that the erupting tooth is a foreign invader), but if the immune system is able to prevent any secondary infection such as ear, chest, or sinus, the battle has been won. Going to the doctor and leaving without a prescription for antibiotics is a sign of a strong immune system, and also that your child is suffering from a virus. That means the body is dealing with the sickness and isn't allowing it to become a bacterial issue. We still want to feed our immune soldiers with the nutrients they need to carry out the battle. Everyone in the family should include the following foods in his or her diet and think about taking some extras in supplement form.

Vitamins A and C

Think reds, oranges, and yellows. Try to eat a variety of colourful fruits and vegetables—they have antioxidants that fight disease, help wounds heal, and support the immune system. Adults should take at least 2000 mg of vitamin C per day—more if you're getting sick—and toddlers between 200 and 400 mg per day in divided doses. This is in addition to what's consumed in the diet. The only side effect of taking too much vitamin C is gas or diarrhea (handy for constipation!).

Zinc and Iron

Zinc and iron are needed for healthy immune function and red blood cells. Good sources of iron and zinc include meat, especially organ meats; seafood, particularly oysters and herring; beans; sunflower and pumpkin seeds; whole grains like oats, amaranth, quinoa, and brown rice; lentils, dried fruit such as figs; blackstrap molasses; mushrooms; green leafy vegetables; kelp; beets; asparagus; avocados; cucumbers; parsley; and bananas. Iron should not be supplemented unless deficiency is diagnosed by blood test. A symptom of zinc deficiency is white marks on the fingernails. If you notice this, a supplement is necessary to correct the deficiency. Gammadyn zinc liquid provides a safe level for anyone (see the Resources section).

Probiotics

With over 80 percent of our immune system found in our digestive system, ensuring a healthy amount of friendly bacteria or probiotics in the digestive tract will boost the immune system (see Chapter 7). At the first sign of any sickness, take an increased amount. Or even better, take an increased level all winter long. If antibiotics are prescribed, keep taking probiotics, and triple the amount after the course has finished.

Raw Garlic

Raw garlic is a superpower! It inhibits the common cold virus, promotes the growth of healthy intestinal flora, and eliminates "bad" bacteria and yeasts. For the common cold, sore throats, and sinus headaches, add raw garlic to anything. For a cure-all garlic remedy, boil a cup of water and add lemon juice to taste and a teaspoon of honey. Using a garlic press, squeeze in one clove garlic, and drink the whole mug. For your toddler, share your mug or tip a bit into her own mug, and encourage drinking the garlic too. Do this a few times a day, and you'll be better in no time (and don't worry about smelling of garlic— you won't see anyone anyway, as you're at home with your toddler).

> ### From the Mouths of Moms: My Story
>
> When my second daughter was getting colds one after the other, she needed a big boost. For a whole month, I gave her fresh banana, avocado, blueberry, and pear purée (see the recipe on page 178) with a clove of raw garlic every day. It killed whatever was hanging around, and she was well for months after. I had lots of comments, though, about her garlic breath!

A drop of garlic oil in the ear canal once a day helps clear ear infections. To prepare the oil, crush several cloves of garlic and soak in ¼ cup (25 mL) olive oil for at least an hour and up to three days. Then strain the oil through cheesecloth, or drain off a few drops of the oil with a dropper (no garlic, just oil), drop into the ear canal, and seal with a bit of cotton wool. Repeat as needed.

Protein

The amino acids in protein are the building blocks of the cells in your immune system, and they help create protective white blood cells and antibodies. Choose lean protein from the following sources: fish, chicken, turkey, eggs, beans, whole grains, legumes, quinoa, tempeh, nuts, and seeds. My family's favourite meal when the girls are sick is a boiled egg and soldiers (toast cut up into finger strips). When I make it for dinner, they feel special. If you can't get food into your toddler, try a smoothie with hemp protein powder in a sippy cup with the valve taken out.

Echinacea

Echinacea is known as a herbal antibiotic that helps boost the immune system. Echinacea works best at the beginning of a cold. If you're already sick, it's not as effective. Long-term use isn't advised as it loses its effectiveness; use it for five days to one week, and then take a break for the same amount of time. Liquid echinacea for children is readily available at supplement and health food stores.

Boiron's Coryzalia

Coryzalia, by Boiron Laboratories, is a homeopathic remedy for babies from 6 to 36 months of age (I used it for my daughters from 2 months) that helps relieve nasal congestion and runny nose. Homeopathy is completely safe for pregnancy and breastfeeding mothers.

Castor Oil

Castor oil, rubbed on the chest, front, and back before bed, helps boost the immune system and "drain" the respiratory system. It's a simple and effective remedy that works especially well with coughing. The oil can also be rubbed over the neck for a sore throat and from the back of the neck up to the back of the ear to help drain the ear canal. It's good, too, for helping to alleviate constipation when rubbed on the abdomen.

TODDLER TIMES RECIPES

ALMOND MILK

I recommend making your own almond milk, as commercial milks can be high in sugar and additives and don't provide nearly the same benefits as whole almonds. If you're feeding your child almond milk, you'll need to add a couple tablespoons of full-fat coconut milk to increase the amount of saturated fat and calories so its nutritional profile is more like that of cow's or goat's milk.

1 cup	raw almonds, preferably organic	250 mL
4 cups	filtered water	1 L
¼ cup	sesame seeds (optional)	50 mL
¼ cup	full-fat coconut milk*	50 mL
2 tsp	agave syrup	10 mL

1. Soak almonds in a bowl of water overnight, or for at least 4 hours. Drain and rinse several times (skip soaking if you're in a rush).
2. In a blender, combine almonds, water, sesame seeds (if using), coconut milk, and agave syrup. Blend for 4 to 5 minutes. Strain with a fine-mesh strainer lined with cheesecloth, a bag for making jelly, or a cloth milk bag (used for nut milks).
3. Keep milk refrigerated in a sealed glass container for up to 2 or 3 days. It can also be frozen. Makes approximately 4 cups (1 L).

* Shake the can thoroughly before opening. Freeze leftover coconut milk in ice cube trays for later use.

NUTRITIONAL INFORMATION
Almonds are a very good source of vitamin E, omega-6 fatty acids, calcium, manganese, magnesium, copper, riboflavin (vitamin B2), and phosphorus. Sesame seeds are a powerhouse of calcium—they contain a much higher level than is found in milk.

LOVELY SOAKED MUESLI

Soaking the grains and seeds releases enzymes that make them easier to digest. A quick, delicious, and nutritious breakfast!

1 cup	oats	250 mL
1 cup	quinoa flakes	250 mL
½ cup	mixed seeds (flax, sunflower, and pumpkin)	125 mL
¼ cup	chopped dried apricots	50 mL
¼ cup	chopped raisins	50 mL
Handful	chopped dried fruit, nuts, or seeds that you like	Handful

1. Combine all ingredients and store in an airtight container in the fridge or freezer.
2. To prepare, put a handful of dry mixture into a bowl. Grate in some apple and cover with your milk of choice. Cover the bowl and refrigerate overnight.
3. Add extra fresh fruit and milk before serving. Makes about 3 cups (750 mL) of dry muesli mix.

NUTRITIONAL INFORMATION
A good source of manganese, selenium, iron, vitamin B1, fibre, magnesium, protein, phosphorus, vitamin C, and zinc.

Your Own Boxed Cereal

Nothing but good stuff in this cereal! This doubles as a great finger food snack—simply leave out the millet puffs and ground nuts and seeds, as they're too hard for little fingers to pick up.

1 cup	Nature's Path Millet Rice Flakes	250 mL
3/4 cup	Barbara's Breakfast O's	175 mL
3/4 cup	Nature's Path Rice Puffs	175 mL
1/2 cup	Nature's Path Millet Puffs	125 mL
1/2 cup	raisins	125 mL
1/2 cup	ground nuts and seeds, or chopped dried fruit	125 mL

1. Mix all ingredients together and store in airtight container or bag. To serve, add milk or eat dry as a snack. Makes about 3 ½ cups (875 mL).

NUTRITIONAL INFORMATION
In addition to being organic, this cereal is gluten free, making it easy to digest; it's also low in salt and made with natural fruit sugars.

SUPER TODDLER SMOOTHIE

Smoothies are a great way to get lots of nutrients into your toddler. Stir in fish oil to add beneficial DHA.

½ cup	milk of choice	125 mL
¼ cup	frozen wild blueberries	50 mL
½	banana	½
¼	pear, cored	¼
1 tbsp	hemp and/or rice protein	15 mL
2 tsp	flax oil	10 mL
2 tsp	molasses (optional)	10 mL
Small handful	sunflower sprouts or raw spinach leaves	Small handful

1. Blend all ingredients in a blender until smooth. Serve immediately. Makes about ¾ cup (175 mL).

NUTRITIONAL INFORMATION

This smoothie is a good source of fibre, antioxidants, and omega-3 fats, as well as protein that will keep your baby going longer.

BEAN BURGERS

Easy for little hands to pick up, these burgers are also great dipped in Apple Butter Dip, hummus, or tzatziki. Serve with Sweet Potato Fries—yummy!

2	carrots	2
1	small onion	1
1	clove garlic	1
Handful	fresh cilantro and/or parsley, chopped	Handful
3 cups	mixed canned chickpeas, kidney beans, and adzuki beans	750 mL
1 tbsp	extra-virgin olive oil	15 mL
1 ½ cups	bread crumbs*	375 mL
2 to 3	eggs	2 to 3

1. In a food processor, pulse carrots, onion, garlic, and cilantro until finely chopped. Add beans and olive oil, and pulse until combined.
2. Add breadcrumbs and 2 eggs and combine thoroughly. If mixture is too dry, add another egg. Let sit for a few minutes.
3. Form into 24 small patties or sausage shapes. Brush a nonstick grill or frying pan with olive oil; heat over medium heat. Cook patties about 5 minutes per side until golden brown, or bake at 350°F (180°C) for 15 minutes, turning once. Suitable for freezing. Makes about 24 mini burgers.

* You can substitute ½ cup (125 mL) ground seeds (sunflower and/or pumpkin) for ½ cup (125 mL) of the bread crumbs.

NUTRITIONAL INFORMATION

A good source of fibre, protein, magnesium, potassium, iron, zinc, copper, manganese, and vitamin B3.

SWEET POTATO FRIES

The trick with these fries is to put loads of garlic and paprika on them. They'll be an instant hit, and you'll love that they're baked, not fried, and contain no salt.

2	medium sweet potatoes or yams, peeled*	2
2 tbsp	extra-virgin olive oil	30 mL
1 tbsp	garlic powder	15 mL
1 tbsp	paprika	15 mL

1. Cut sweet potatoes into small fries either by hand or with a mandolin. In a sealed storage bag, toss the sweet potato fries with olive oil, garlic, and paprika, coating completely.

2. Spread out on a parchment-lined baking tray and bake at 350°F (180°C) for 20 minutes or until tender (they won't be as crispy as potato fries). Makes 2 to 4 servings.

* You can also keep the skin on. Parsnips, carrots, or potatoes are also good.

NUTRITIONAL INFORMATION
Sweet potatoes are high in beta carotene, fibre, potassium, and vitamins C and E.

SMARTY PANTS FISH CAKES

A great way to introduce fish, if you haven't already. Serve these with Apple Butter Dip.

1 lb	potatoes, peeled	500 g
1	clove garlic, peeled and chopped in half	1
¼ cup	frozen corn	50 mL
¼ cup	frozen peas	50 mL
¼ lb	fish fillet of your choice*	125 g
2 heaping tbsp	chopped fresh dill or cilantro	30 mL
1 cup	gluten-free breadcrumbs or sesame seeds	250 mL

1. Chop potatoes into small cubes. Add with garlic to a medium saucepan of boiling water and cook until tender, 7 to 10 minutes. Drain and mash in a large bowl. Stir in frozen corn and peas (hot potatoes will defrost them). Let cool for 5 minutes.
2. Bake fish at 400°F (200°C) for 10 to 12 minutes or until flaky.
3. Place fish on top of mashed potato mixture; add dill and gently mix together. Don't overmix as potatoes can become gluey. Form mixture into burger or finger shapes and coat with breadcrumbs or sesame seeds, shaking off excess. Fish cakes are cooked and ready to eat—serve immediately or warm in a frying pan or oven later.
4. Suitable for freezing. Makes about 12 to 16 fish cakes.

* White fish such as cod is mild tasting and best for new fish eaters, but wild salmon is excellent here. You can substitute 5.3 oz (150 g) canned fish, drained, for fresh. For more EFAs, use canned wild salmon.

NUTRITIONAL INFORMATION
A very good source of protein, omega-3 fats (if using salmon), vitamin C, vitamin B6, copper, potassium, manganese, and fibre.

APPLE BUTTER DIP

This dip is fabulous with the bean burgers and fish cakes above. It's a versatile sauce that can be used in both sweet and savoury dishes. I like to turn this into a stir-fry sauce by adding grated ginger and extra lemon and garlic. It's also delicious as a topping for roasted salmon.

1 cup	apple butter (I recommend Filsinger's)	250 mL
2	cloves garlic, finely chopped	2
2 tbsp	lemon juice	30 mL
2 tsp	extra-virgin olive oil	10 mL

1. Stir together all ingredients. Can be stored in the refrigerator for up to 3 weeks. Makes about 1 cup (250 mL).

NUTRITIONAL INFORMATION
A healthy fruit sauce that contains no sugar. Garlic is antibacterial and antiviral, and therefore boosts the immune system. Apple butter contains fibre and flavonoids.

VEGGIE-PACKED CHILI

Veggie chili is a staple for the whole family. Feel free to add other veggies than those listed here. Serve with brown rice or baked potato.

1 tbsp	extra-virgin olive oil	15 mL
1	onion, chopped	1
1	clove garlic, chopped	1
1	small eggplant or zucchini, chopped	1
1	head cauliflower, chopped	1
2	carrots, chopped	2
½	red pepper, chopped	½
Handful	shiitake or button mushrooms	Handful
1 tsp	chili powder	5 mL
1	can (28 oz/796 mL) diced tomatoes*	1
1	can (14 oz/398 mL) kidney beans, drained and rinsed	1
3 tbsp	chopped fresh parsley	45 mL

1. Heat olive oil in a large saucepan. Add onion and garlic and sauté until soft. Add eggplant or zucchini, cauliflower, carrots, red pepper, mushrooms, and chili powder; sauté for a few minutes.
2. Add tomatoes and bring to a boil. Reduce heat and simmer for 20 minutes. Stir in kidney beans and parsley and cook for another 10 minutes.
3. Serve over baked potato, rice, or noodles and top with grated cheese. Makes about 6 cups (1.5 L).

* To avoid potential BPA in canned tomatoes, substitute a 24 oz (739 mL) jar of tomato sauce and ¼ cup water.

NUTRITIONAL INFORMATION
A good source of molybdenum, folate, fibre, manganese, protein, thiamine (vitamin B1), phosphorus, iron, copper, magnesium, potassium, and vitamin K.

TODDLER 12 MONTHS+ MEAL PLANNER

Offer water throughout the day. Some moms may continue to breastfeed upon rising and at bedtime.

	Upon Rising	Breakfast	Snack	Lunch	Snack	Dinner	Bedtime
Day 1	Milk*	Amazing Sweet Amaranth (not puréed)	Dried fruit with cheese	Introduction to Lentils over brown rice pasta Milk before nap	Rice cake with apple butter and almond butter	Veggie-Packed Chili with baked potato	Milk
Day 2	Milk	Finger Food Pancakes and Super Toddler Smoothie	Rice cake and hummus	Bean and Rice Surprise (not puréed) Milk before nap	Yogurt with Spiced-Up Apples or Pears	Bean Burgers and Sweet Potato Fries	Milk
Day 3	Milk	Lovely Soaked Muesli	Apple slices and almond butter	Leftover Bean Burger patties with carrot sticks and hummus Milk before nap	Rice cake with Yummy Carrot Spread	Fish cakes with Apple Butter Dip and steamed veggie sticks	Milk

Milk: Full-fat, organic, cow's, goat's, sheep's, or homemade almond milk (see recipe p. 231)

TASTES FOR TODDLERS 18 MONTHS+

Veggie Pesto Pizza

Pizza is a great way to sneak in a ton of vegetables. Stack it thick, and whatever vegetables fall on the plate will be picked up by little fingers. The unbaked assembled pizza can be frozen.

PESTO:	2 cups	packed fresh basil leaves	500 mL
	½ cup	packed fresh cilantro leaves	125 mL
	2 tbsp	sunflower seeds	30 mL
	2 tsp	capers	10 mL
	4	kalamata olives, pitted	4
	4	sundried tomatoes	4
	2	garlic cloves, peeled	2
	⅓ cup	extra-virgin olive oil	75 mL
	Pinch	sea salt	Pinch
	2 small or 1 large	pizza bases (preferably gluten free or spelt)	2 small or 1 large
	1 cup	shredded goat's or cow's milk mozzarella cheese	250 mL

SUGGESTED PIZZA TOPPINGS (FINELY CHOPPED):

Green beans, corn, asparagus, shiitake or button mushrooms, onions, broccoli, red or yellow peppers, spinach, raisins

1. To make the pesto: In a food processor, combine basil, cilantro, sunflower seeds, capers, olives, sundried tomatoes, and garlic; pulse a few times. Slowly add the olive oil in a constant stream while the food processor is running. Stop to scrape down the sides with a rubber spatula. Add a pinch of salt to taste.
2. Top pizza bases with a layer of pesto. Sprinkle with 2 tbsp (30 mL) of the cheese and scatter with toppings, covering all edges. Make it colourful and press the vegetables firmly onto the crust. Top with remaining cheese.
3. Bake at 400°F (200°C) about 15 to 20 minutes or until cheese is melted and crust is crisp. Makes 2 small or 1 large pizza.

NUTRITIONAL INFORMATION
A good source of fibre, protein, vitamin K, iron, calcium, and vitamin A.

LENTIL SHEPHERD'S PIE

This recipe is well loved in my family. A hearty and delicious meal that even meat eaters will enjoy.

½ cup	dried green or French lentils	120 mL
1	slice kombu seaweed	1
1 ½ lb	potatoes*	681 g
1 tbsp	butter	15 mL
1 tbsp	milk	15 mL
1 tbsp	olive oil	15 mL
1	large onion, chopped	1
1	garlic clove, minced	1
2	carrots, peeled and diced	2
¾ cup	chopped button or shiitake mushrooms	175 mL
½ cup	peas	125 mL
1 ¾ cups	tomato (pasta) sauce	425 mL
1 tbsp	tamari	15 mL
1 bunch	parsley, chopped	1 bunch

1. Place the lentils in a medium-sized saucepan, cover with water, and add kombu. Simmer for 45 minutes or until soft. Discard kombu, drain lentils, and set aside.
2. While the lentils are cooking, boil the potatoes until tender. Drain and mash with the butter and milk.
3. Heat the oil in a saucepan over medium heat, and sauté the onions and garlic until transparent. Add carrots and cook for 5 minutes. Add mushrooms and peas and sauté for 2 minutes. Stir in tomato sauce, tamari, half of the parsley, and the cooked lentils. Cook for a few more minutes and remove from heat.
4. Pour the lentil mixture into an oven-proof dish and top with mashed potatoes. Sprinkle with remaining parsley.
   Freeze, or if eating immediately, bake for 30 minutes at 375°F (190°C), or until the potato is golden brown. Makes 6 to 8 servings.

* Parsnip or yam can be substituted for some of the potato.

NUTRITIONAL INFORMATION
A good source of molybdenum, folate, fibre, manganese, iron, protein, phosphorus, copper, thiamine, and potassium.

SWEET POTATO AND COCONUT SOUP

This appetizing soup, bursting with flavour and vitamin C, makes a lovely accompaniment. It can be served as a main meal with whole grain bread or by adding in cooked brown rice.

4 cups	low-sodium vegetable or chicken broth	1 L
2	sweet potatoes, peeled and chopped	2
½ cup	red lentils, rinsed well	125 mL
1	onion, chopped	1
1	kale leaf, chopped	1
1	clove garlic, chopped	1
2 tsp	ground cumin	10 mL
1 ½ tsp	ground coriander	7 mL
1 ½ tsp	chopped fresh ginger root	7 mL
1	can (14 oz/398 mL) coconut milk	1
1 tbsp	chopped fresh cilantro	15 mL

1. Combine broth, sweet potatoes, lentils, onion, kale, garlic, cumin, coriander, and ginger root in a large saucepan and bring to a boil. Turn down heat and simmer, uncovered, until sweet potato is tender, about 20 minutes.
2. Stir in coconut milk and cilantro and purée until smooth. Makes about 6 cups (1.5 L).

NUTRITIONAL INFORMATION
A good source of beta carotene, fibre, potassium, manganese, and vitamins C and E.

SAVOURY AMARANTH WITH VEGETABLES

A twist on the standard rice stir-fry. Packed full of calcium and protein.

2 cups	low-sodium chicken or vegetable stock	500 mL
2 tsp	agave syrup	10 mL
1 cup	amaranth, toasted in a dry frying pan until it pops	250 mL
2 tsp	coconut oil	10 mL
½	onion, finely chopped	½
½ cup	chopped broccoli	125 mL
½ cup	chopped button mushrooms	125 mL
½	red pepper, chopped	½
1	clove garlic, chopped	1
2 tsp	sesame oil	10 mL
1 tsp	tamari	5 mL

1. In a medium saucepan, combine the stock and agave syrup and bring to a boil. Add the toasted amaranth and simmer until all the water has been absorbed, 7 to 10 minutes.
2. Heat coconut oil in a frying pan and add onion, cooking until transparent. Add broccoli, mushrooms, red pepper, and garlic and stir-fry for about 5 minutes or until soft. Stir in cooked amaranth and cook for about 2 minutes longer. Toss with sesame oil and tamari and serve. Makes about 6 servings.

NUTRITIONAL INFORMATION
A good source of folic acid, calcium, protein, vitamin C, and vitamin E.

Super Chicken Burgers, Meatballs, or Meatloaf

This is the perfect place to hide lots of vegetables. Use a variety of vegetables, especially those that you wouldn't normally serve on their own.

1 ½ lb	organic fresh ground chicken or turkey	750 g
2 ½ cups	mixed vegetables,* finely chopped	625 g
1 cup	gluten-free breadcrumbs	250 g
1	onion, diced	1
3	cloves garlic, minced	3
1	egg**	1
Pinch	Salt and pepper	Pinch

1. Combine ingredients in a large bowl and mix thoroughly with your hands. The texture should be sticky, and the mixture should hold its shape. Form into burger shapes or meatballs, or pat into a mini loaf pan. Makes about 3 mini loaves and 12 meatballs or mini burgers.

2. For meatballs: Cook on a parchment-lined baking tray in a 350°F (180°C) oven for 15 to 20 minutes, or until internal temperature reaches 165°F (74°C). Can also be pan fried for 15 minutes until golden brown and cooked through.
   For meat loaf: Bake for approximately 30 minutes at 350°F (180°C) or until internal temperature reaches 165°F (74°C).
   For burgers: Freeze raw by placing individual burgers on a parchment-lined baking tray. Once frozen, transfer to freezer bag for storage. To cook, barbecue or fry in a skillet over medium-high heat until brown on each side and internal temperature reaches 165°F (74°C).

*Mixed vegetables can include (choose 3 or 4 options):
Zucchini, kale, red or yellow peppers, broccoli, carrot, green beans, green peas, corn, parsley, cilantro, swiss chard, apple

** If you wish to omit the egg, decrease the amount of breadcrumbs to ½ cup (125 mL).

NUTRITIONAL INFORMATION
A good source of protein, fibre, and nutrients.

LASAGNA

A great weekend recipe to make in a large batch and freeze for future meals. The sauce is another good place to sneak veggies into.

6 to 8	sheets rice or kamut lasagna noodles	6 to 8
2 tbsp	olive oil	30 mL
1	small onion, chopped	1
1 to 2	cloves garlic, chopped	1 to 2
1 lb	ground organic dark meat chicken or turkey	500 g
1	jar (24 oz/739 mL) tomato sauce*	1
½ cup	water	125 mL
1	red or yellow pepper, chopped	1
2	carrots, chopped	2
½ cup	chopped button or shiitake mushrooms	125 mL
2 tbsp	chopped fresh parsley	30 mL
1 tbsp	Italian seasoning	15 mL
Handful	spinach leaves, washed	Handful
1 ½ cups	shredded organic mozzarella cheese	375 mL

1. Cook lasagna noodles in boiling water until tender (don't overcook as they fall apart). Drain, drizzle with 1 tablespoon of the olive oil (so they don't stick), and place on a parchment-lined baking tray. Cover with damp tea towels.

2. Heat remaining olive oil in a large saucepan and cook onion and garlic until transparent. Mix in ground chicken and brown. Stir in tomato sauce, water, red pepper, carrots, mushrooms, parsley, and Italian seasoning. Cook for about 20 minutes or until carrots are soft.

3. Use 3 loaf pans or a 13- by 9-inch baking dish. Spread a tablespoon of sauce in the bottom of pan, then layer noodles, meat sauce, spinach, and cheese, repeating layers until the pan is full. Freeze until needed.

4. Defrost overnight in the fridge, then bake in 350°F (180°C) oven for about 30 to 45 minutes (depending on size) until heated through.

*Jarred tomato sauce doesn't potentially contain bisphenol A as canned tomatoes do.

NUTRITIONAL INFORMATION
A nutrient-rich meal containing antioxidants, calcium, magnesium, iron, zinc, and vitamin C. Also a balanced meal of protein, carbohydrate, and vegetables.

BEAN AND VEGGIE KAMUT QUESADILLAS

A crowd pleaser! Feel free to substitute any of your toddler's favourite veggies. All measurements are estimated—add more of whatever you like.

1 cup	adzuki, kidney, and/or cannellini beans, drained and rinsed	250 mL
½	red pepper, diced	½
½ cup	corn, chopped if necessary	125 mL
½ cup	finely chopped broccoli	125 mL
½ cup	chopped cooked chicken (optional)	125 mL
6	kamut wraps*	6
1 cup	shredded goat's milk mozzarella cheese	250 mL

1. Combine beans, red pepper, corn, broccoli, and chicken (if using) in a bowl.
2. Heat a frying pan over medium-high heat. Place a wrap in the pan; sprinkle with some cheese and top with the bean mixture. Sprinkle with a little more cheese and top with another wrap. Press down firmly with your hands or a spatula and cook until crisp. Flip and cook until crisp, the filling is heated through, and cheese has melted. Serve with salsa or guacamole. Makes 3 to 4 quesadillas.

* Whole grain wraps or corn tortillas can be substituted.

NUTRITIONAL INFORMATION
Contains fibre, vitamin C, calcium, protein, and beta carotene.

CRISPY CHICKEN NIBBLES

While the chicken is cooking, make the Apple Butter Dip above, a great alternative to ketchup or plum sauce.

2	skinless, boneless chicken breasts	2
1 cup	gluten-free breadcrumbs	250 mL
1 to 2 tsp	mixed dried herbs (basil, oregano, thyme)	5 to 10 mL
1 tsp	garlic powder	5 mL
2	large eggs	2
½ cup	flour (any type)	125 mL

1. Cut chicken into strips or small pieces.
2. Mix breadcrumbs, herbs, and garlic powder together in a bowl. Whisk eggs in a shallow dish and place flour in another shallow dish. Coat chicken in flour, then dip into egg, coating evenly and shaking off excess. Press chicken into breadcrumb mixture to coat. Transfer to a plate and repeat with remaining chicken.
3. Heat a nonstick frying pan over medium heat. Cook chicken for about 7 to 15 minutes (depending on size), turning once, until golden brown and cooked through. Makes 2 to 3 servings.

NUTRITIONAL INFORMATION
A good source of protein.

SPROUT RIGHT'S DIVINE COOKIES

Nobody will guess there's no sugar in these cookies—they're truly divine!

1 cup	unsalted butter, at room temperature	250 mL
2 ½ tsp	vanilla	12 mL
1	egg	1
¼ cup plus 2 ½ tbsp	agave syrup	87 mL
1 ½ cups	brown rice flour	375 mL
¼ cup	potato starch	50 mL
¼ cup	tapioca starch	50 mL
¾ tsp	baking powder	4 mL
½ tsp	salt	2 mL
¼ tsp	xanthan gum	1 mL

Shredded coconut, or chopped nuts (optional)

Unsweetened jam or apple butter

1. In a mixer beat butter, vanilla, and egg. Pour in the agave syrup and beat; mixture will look curdled. Add in the dry ingredients and mix thoroughly. If possible, let batter stand for 10 minutes at room temperature.

2. Drop dough by spoonfuls onto parchment-lined baking tray, or form into balls and roll in nuts or shredded coconut (if using). Use your finger to make an indentation in the centre and fill with jam or apple butter.

3. Bake in a 325°F (160°C) oven for 15 to 18 minutes or until golden brown around the edges. Let stand two minutes; transfer to a rack to cool. Makes 18 to 24 cookies.

NUTRITIONAL INFORMATION
A healthy cookie made without gluten or sugar. Contains protein, iron, and potassium.

SNEAKY LITTLE MUFFINS

These muffins make tasty snacks. I like to make and freeze a batch to defrost for an accompaniment to lunch or a snack on car rides.

2	overripe bananas	2
2	eggs	2
1 cup	grated carrots	250 mL
½ cup	agave syrup	125 mL
½ cup	rice milk	125 mL
6 tbsp	melted butter	90 mL
¼ cup	grated zucchini	50 mL
⅓ cup	ground chia (Salba)	75 mL
1 ¾ cup	brown rice flour	425 mL
¼ cup	tapioca starch	50 mL
2 tsp	baking powder	10 mL
1 tsp	baking soda	5 mL
1 tsp	cinnamon	5 mL

1. Beat the bananas in a mixer. Beat in eggs. Add carrots, agave syrup, rice milk, butter, zucchini, and chia; mix well and let sit for 5 minutes.

2. In another bowl, stir together rice flour, tapioca, baking powder, baking soda, and cinnamon. Add dry ingredients to wet ingredients and mix thoroughly.

3. Spoon into 36 greased or paper-lined mini muffin cups and bake in 325°F (160°C) oven for about 25 minutes or until muffins are golden and lightly spring back when touched. Makes about 36 mini muffins.

NUTRITIONAL INFORMATION
A healthy gluten-free, sugar-free, dairy-free snack containing beta carotene, potassium, fibre, protein, and trace minerals.

SINLESS CHOCOLATE ALMOND BROWNIES

With dark chocolate, gluten-free flour, natural alternatives to sugar, and even goat's milk butter, this unique recipe will ease your guilt and offer some power-packed nutrition as well. Although not as sweet as what you might be accustomed to, these brownies are quite addictive! You can easily substitute unsalted butter for the goat's milk butter, or cane sugar for the brown rice syrup.

3 oz	dark chocolate (at least 70% cocoa solids)	85 g
2 tbsp	goat's milk butter	30 g
½ cup	brown rice syrup	125 mL
2	large organic eggs	2
1 tsp	pure vanilla extract	5 mL
½ cup	gluten-free flour mix (e.g., Bob's Red Mill)	125 mL
½ cup	chopped almonds (optional)	125 mL

1. Melt the chocolate and butter in a medium-sized saucepan over low heat. Stir in the brown rice syrup and remove from heat. Whisk in the eggs one at a time, and add the vanilla. Stir in the flour and nuts (if using).

2. Pour the mixture into greased, parchment paper-lined, 8-inch (2 L) square baking pan and spread evenly. Bake in a 350°F (180°C) oven for 20 to 25 minutes or until just set. Turn out onto a cooling rack and cut into squares. Store in an airtight container, if they last that long! Makes about 16 brownies.

NUTRITIONAL INFORMATION
Dark chocolate is high in magnesium and contains an abundant amount of antioxidants. Almonds are high in calcium, magnesium, vitamin E, and fibre.

APPLE CRUMBLE

This is a recipe based on my mom's apple crumble. I've made it healthier while keeping it scrumptious.

3 cups	sliced fruit: apples, peaches, pears, or a combo	750 mL
1 cup	blueberries or other berries	250 mL
¼ cup	100% fruit juice	50 mL
1 tsp	cinnamon	5 mL
CRUMBLE TOPPING:		
1 ½ cups	rolled oats	375 mL
¼ cup	maple syrup (or agave)	50 mL
¼ cup	sunflower seeds, chopped	50 mL
¼ cup	walnuts, chopped	50 mL
¼ cup	unsalted butter	50 mL
1 tsp	cinnamon	5 mL

1. In a bowl, toss the sliced fruit, blueberries, fruit juice, and cinnamon.
2. In another bowl, mix the oats, syrup, sunflower seeds, walnuts, butter, and cinnamon. Rub between your fingers to create a soft, coarse crumble.
3. Spoon the fruit mixture and its liquid into a pie plate. Top with the crumble mixture and bake in a 350°F (180°C) oven for 35 to 45 minutes, or until the fruit is fork tender and the filling is bubbling and thickened (can also be frozen before cooked). The top should be golden brown. Cool slightly on a wire rack before serving warm or at room temperature. Makes 6 to 8 servings.

NUTRITIONAL INFORMATION
Rich in vitamin C, fibre, antioxidants, essential fatty acids, trace minerals, and complex carbohydrates.

Organic Rice Crisp Surprise Squares

Adults and kids alike will find these hard to resist.

½ cup	brown rice syrup	125 mL
2 tbsp	blackstrap molasses	30 mL
¼ cup	almond butter	50 mL
1/8 cup	tahini	25 mL
1/8 cup	sunflower seed butter	25 mL
1 tsp	vanilla	5 mL
½ box	Barbara's Organic Rice Crisps	140 g
1/8 cup	sunflower seeds	25 mL
1/8 cup	pumpkin seeds	25 mL

1. Heat rice syrup, molasses, almond butter, tahini, sunflower seed butter, and vanilla in a saucepan over medium-low heat until well combined and almost runny. Remove from heat.
2. Add cereal, sunflower seeds, and pumpkin seeds and quickly stir well to coat. Press into two 8-inch (2 L) square trays and let cool. Makes about 32 to 64 squares, depending on how small you cut them.

NUTRITIONAL INFORMATION
A good source of vitamin E, calcium, zinc, vitamin B1, manganese, magnesium, copper, selenium, phosphorus, vitamin B5, and folate.

GO FASTER GRANOLA BARS

These wholesome granola bars are packed with slow-releasing carbohydrates and healthy fats to keep your toddler going longer.

1 cup	Nature's Path Millet Rice Flakes cereal	250 mL
1 cup	whole rolled oats	250 mL
3/4 cup	dried fruit (raisins, chopped dates, apricots)	175 mL
1/4 cup	sunflower, pumpkin, or sesame seeds	50 mL
1/4 cup	chopped almonds	50 mL
1/2 cup	brown rice syrup	125 mL
2 tbsp	coconut butter or unsalted butter	30 mL
1/4 cup	almond butter	50 mL

1. Mix cereal flakes, rolled oats, dried fruit, seeds, and almonds in a bowl.
2. Gently heat brown rice syrup, coconut butter, and almond butter in a large saucepan until melted and smooth. Add dry ingredients to saucepan and quickly stir well to coat. Press into an 8-inch (2 L) square pan.
3. Refrigerate for at least 1 hour and cut into squares. Store at room temperature. Makes about 16 bars.

NUTRITIONAL INFORMATION
A good source of vitamin E, calcium, zinc, vitamin B1, manganese, magnesium, protein, copper, selenium, phosphorus, vitamin B5, and folate.

No-Mess Fruity Pops

A refreshing summer treat, loaded with nutrients.

4 cups	fresh fruit salad*	1 L
½ cup	applesauce (optional)	125 mL

1. Blend fruit salad in a blender or food processor until smooth. If you want to stretch it more, add applesauce. Pour purée into popsicle moulds and freeze. Makes about 4 popsicles.

* Banana, peach, pear, blueberry, and mango are a good combination, but any fruit will work well.

NUTRITIONAL INFORMATION
A good source of fibre, antioxidants, and vitamin C.

Fruity Frozen Yogurt

Your kids will think they're being spoiled when they eat this! A delightfully healthy yet tasty treat.

1 cup	yogurt	250 mL
2 ½ cups	fruit salad*	625 mL
½	ripe avocado (optional)	½
3 tbsp	maple syrup or honey	45 mL

1. Divide yogurt among ice cube trays and freeze. Spread fruit salad evenly on a parchment-lined baking tray and freeze.
2. Once frozen, take yogurt out of the freezer for 3 to 5 minutes to soften slightly. Purée yogurt, frozen fruit, avocado, and maple syrup in a food processor until smooth. Makes about 2 cups (500 mL).

* Be sure to include banana for sweetness and creamy texture.

NUTRITIONAL INFORMATION
A good source of calcium, phosphorus, vitamin B2, protein, vitamin B12, potassium, molybdenum, zinc, and pantothenic acid.

TODDLER 18 MONTHS+ MEAL PLANNER

Offer water throughout the day. Some moms may continue to breastfeed upon rising and at bedtime.

	Upon Rising	Breakfast	Snack	Lunch	Snack	Dinner	Bedtime
Day 1	Milk*	Toast and eggs and Super Toddler Smoothie	Apple slices with cheese	Veggie Pesto Pizza	Rice cake with fruit spread and almond butter	Super Chicken Burger with Sweet Potato Fries and steamed broccoli	Milk
Day 2	Milk	Oatmeal (with cinnamon and chopped fruit)	Rice cake and hummus	Leftover chicken burger made into a wrap with sprouts and apple butter	Yogurt with Spiced-Up Apples or Pears	Sweet Potato and Coconut Soup with whole grain bread and hummus	Milk
Day 3	Milk	Your Own Boxed Cereal and scrambled eggs	Apple slices and almond butter	Leftover soup with veggie sticks and hummus	Veggie sticks with Beany Green Dip	Lasagna and slices of fresh peppers	Milk

Milk: Full-fat, organic, cow's, goat's, or homemade almond milk (see recipe p. 242)

Resources

Supplements

The following are supplements made by reputable companies. Note that supplement companies often change their formulations or product names and sometimes discontinue items. Consult with a nutritionist or naturopath before deciding which is right for you.

Genestra

Pregna Vit—pre- and postnatal vitamin/mineral supplement. Take three capsules with breakfast. Extra folic acid may be required in some cases.

Cal Mag Liquid—useful as an antacid as well as a good calcium and magnesium supplement

Super DHA Liquid—yields 1200 mg DHA per teaspoon

Cod Liver Oil, Super EPA Liquid, and Berry EFA Plus—liquid DHA/EPA—offer different levels of DHA

Super EFA Plus—capsules of EPA/DHA

Super Neurogen DHA—algae DHA only in vegetarian gel cap (vegetarian). Pierce a hole in the capsule and squeeze into baby's mouth.

Neurogen DHA—algae DHA only in capsule (vegan)

Probiotics

HMF Natogen for infants under one year old

HMF Powder for one year and older

HMF Super Powder for yeast or candida symptoms

HMF Forte capsules for adults

HMF Intensive for higher level of good bacteria after illness

HMF Replete for adults or over one year of age after antibiotic therapy

Gammadyn Minerals including zinc—Unda product by Seroyal

D-mulsion—vitamin D drops for baby and adults

Ascorbete C—vitamin C powder for any age (other than newborn)

Echinasyr—echinacea for immune boosting for babies over six months

Thorne—pre- and postnatal, calcium, and magnesium supplements

Metagenics—pre- and postnatal

Nutra Sea—omega-3 fish oils

Nordic Naturals—omega-3 fish oils

Carlson—D drops for mom and baby, cod-liver oil

Platinum Easy Iron—for mom or baby (pierce a hole in the capsule for baby)

Hylands—teething tablets and gel, tissue salts

Schlusser Tissue Salts—tissue salt combinations including "Healthy Appetite"

Boiron—homeopathic remedies for teething, colds, and colic

Pregnancy and Breastfeeding

Motherisk—www.motherisk.org

Ann Douglas, "The Mother of All" book series (Toronto: Wiley).

Jack Newman, *Dr. Jack Newman's Guide to Breastfeeding*, revised ed. (Toronto: HarperCollins, 2003).

William Sears and Martha Sears, *The Baby Book: Everything You Need to Know about Your Baby from Birth to Age Two*, 2nd ed. (Boston: Little, Brown: 2003).

Websites for New Parent Support

www.savvymom.com

www.wccwelcome.ca

www.sweetmama.ca

www.babycentre.ca

www.canadianparents.com

www.todaysparent.ca

www.parentcentral.ca

Lactation Support

Dr. Jack Newman—www.drjacknewman.com

4th trimester—www.4thtrimester.ca

International Lactation Consultant Association—www.ilca.org

La Leche League—www.lllc.ca

Organic Hypericum and Calendula Tincture for cracked nipples—www.nealsyardremedies.com

SLEEP SUPPORT

The Sleep Doula—www.sleepdoula.com

Harvey Karp, *The Happiest Baby on the Block: The New Way to Calm Crying and Help Your Baby Sleep Longer* (New York: Bantam, 2002).

Marc Weissbluth, *Healthy Sleep Habits, Happy Child: A Step-by-Step Program for a Good Night's Sleep* (New York: Ballantine Books, 2005).

FOOD AND PRODUCT SAFETY

Canadian Food Inspection Agency Food Recall Alerts—www.inspection.gc.ca/english/corpaffr/recarapp/recaltoce.shtml

Environmental Working Group's Skin Deep Cosmetics Database—www.cosmeticsdatabase.com

Environmental Working Group—www.ewg.org

Health Canada—www.hc-sc.gc.ca

Institute for Agricultural and Trade Policy Food and Health—www.iatp.org/foodandhealth

U.S. Food and Drug Administration—www.fda.gov

ALLERGIES

Carolee Bateson-Koch, *Allergies: Disease in Disguise* (Burnaby, BC: Alive Books, 2002).

Lucy Burney, *Boost Your Child's Immune System: A Program and Recipes for Raising Strong, Healthy Kids* (New York: Newmarket Press, 2005).

Konrad Kail and Bobbi Lawrence, *Allergy Free: An Alternative Medicine Definitive Guide* (Tiburon, CA: AlternativeMedicine.com Books, 2000).

Doris Rapp, *Is This Your Child? Discovering and Treating Unrecognized Allergies in Children and Adults* (New York: William Morrow and Company, 1991).

HEALTH

Phyllis A. Balch, *Prescription for Dietary Wellness,* 2nd ed. (New York: Avery, 2003).

David Hoffman, *Holistic Herbal* (London: Thorsons, 1990).

Janet Zand, Robert Rountree, and Rachel Walton, *Smart Medicine for a Healthier Child,* 2nd ed. (New York: Penguin, 2003).

WATER

Brita Filters—www.brita.com

Aquareal Water Company—www.aquareal.com

Dasani bottled water—reverse osmosis water

Culligan water service offering large bottles and filter systems—www.culligan.ca

Whole Foods Market and other stores often have self-fill reverse osmosis systems

Food Sources of Vitamins and Minerals

Fat-Soluble Vitamins

Vitamin A

Antioxidant, helps with vision and growth, immune enhancer, supports mucosal membranes such as the lungs. Best absorbed cooked.

Found in: carrots, avocados, spinach, yellow/orange fruits and vegetables (cantaloupe, yams, papaya), dark-green leafy vegetables (watercress, dandelion greens, broccoli, kale), liver, eggs, milk and milk products, cod-liver oil, seaweed, and garlic

Vitamin D

Helps strengthen teeth and bones, essential for normal growth and development, supports the heart and immune system, promotes normal blood clotting, and helps absorption of calcium

Found in: salmon, sardines, herring, tuna, organ meats, cod-liver oil, vitamin D–fortified milk and milk products, egg yolks, wheat germ, and oats

Vitamin E

Antioxidant, maintains healthy skin, strengthens capillary walls, reduces cholesterol, reduces PMS symptoms and menopausal hot flashes, and protects against cancer

Found in: peas, lettuce, sweet potatoes, leafy vegetables, brown rice, rye, whole grain cereals, wheat germ, nuts, egg yolks, organ meats, molasses, corn oil, cold-pressed oils, sunflower seeds, and olives

Vitamin K

Helps with blood clotting and aids in absorption of vitamin D

Found in: alfalfa, green vegetables, chlorophyll, cauliflower, oats, wheat, rye, soybeans, egg yolks, liver, yogurt, acidophilus, safflower oil, and blackstrap molasses

WATER-SOLUBLE VITAMINS

B Vitamins

All B vitamins are essential for energy; growth; body maintenance, including healthy nerves, skin, hair, and eyes; as well as food digestion and metabolism.

VITAMIN B1 (THIAMINE): Breaks down carbohydrates, stabilizes appetite, and regulates nerve impulses

Found in: legumes, wheat germ, brewer's yeast, whole grains, sunflower seeds, nuts, organ meats, fish and poultry, egg yolks, and blackstrap molasses

VITAMIN B2 (RIBOFLAVIN): Essential for growth, breaks down fat and carbohydrate, aids in the absorption of iron from digestive tract, and used by the adrenal glands for hormone production

Found in: carrots, mushrooms, spinach, broccoli, legumes, brussels sprouts, kelp, prunes, apples, lemons, grapefruit, coconut, whole grains, wheat germ, brewer's yeast, nuts, organ meats, egg yolks, milk and milk products, and blackstrap molasses

VITAMIN B3 (NIACIN): Breaks down carbohydrates and fats in body, helps nervous system, reduces cholesterol levels, aids stomach acid production, and promotes growth

Found in: rhubarb, whole barley, avocados, eggs, dates, figs, prunes, wheat germ, whole bran, peanuts, almonds, leafy greens, fish (including lobster), poultry, and milk and milk products

VITAMIN B5 (PANTOTHENIC ACID): Helps to break down carbohydrates and fats, important for adrenal function, helps the use of iron, important for healthy skin and nerves and antibody formation

Found in: broccoli, legumes, whole grains, wheat bran, wheat germ, eggs, sunflower seeds, brewer's yeast, peanuts, organ meats, salmon, and blackstrap molasses

VITAMIN B6 (PYRIDOXINE): Essential for normal growth, needed for healthy red blood cells and absorption of B12, plays a role in cancer prevention, produces stomach acid, aids nervous system, helps with PMS and menopausal symptoms

Found in: legumes, green leafy vegetables, cabbage, prunes, bananas, garlic, cauliflower, seaweed, whole grains, wheat germ, brewer's yeast, organ meats, egg yolks, corn oil, blackstrap molasses, and honey

VITAMIN B12 (CYANOCOBALAMIN): Involved in red blood cell production, helps prevent postpartum depression, helps concentration and memory, stabilizes appetite, and supports nerve function

Found in: saltwater fish, pork, organ meats, seaweed, eggs, milk and milk products, tempeh, miso, and brewer's yeast

FOLIC ACID: Ensures that cells develop normally, promotes healthy red blood cells, fosters hydrochloric acid production, prevents spina bifida in the first trimester, improves lactation, and helps stomach acid production

Found in: dark-green leafy vegetables, root vegetables, dates, starchy vegetables, sweet potatoes, parsnips, peas, legumes, seaweed, cauliflower, cabbage, whole grains, brewer's yeast, salmon, tuna, organ meats, and milk

Vitamin C

Antioxidant, maintains skin tissue, aids iron absorption and the use of folic acid, important in wound healing, provides immune support, builds healthy bones and teeth, promotes collagen production, supports artery repair, and reduces cholesterol levels

Found in: green and red peppers, avocados, banana, cabbage, kiwi, turnip greens, kale, collards, parsley, broccoli, tomatoes, mango, citrus fruits, blackcurrants, berries, pineapple, tomatoes, acerola cherries, cantaloupe, strawberries, kiwi, and rosehips

MINERALS

Calcium

Important for growth of bones and teeth and blood clotting, supports a healthy heart, used in muscle contraction and growth, and buffers high-protein and acidic diets

Found in: green leafy vegetables, avocados, celery, seaweed, carrots, dried fruit, papaya, apricots, almonds, nuts and seeds, garlic, brown rice, dried herbs, seaweed, raisins, amaranth, beans, shellfish, milk and milk products, and molasses

Magnesium

Important for muscle contraction, helps calcium absorption, used in acid/alkaline balance with calcium, supports blood sugar balance, helps the body use B vitamins and vitamin C and E, and encourages proper nerve function

Found in: dark-green vegetables, kelp, pineapple, whole grains, nuts, almonds, pecans, seafood, spinach, tofu, bananas, pumpkin seeds, molasses, and honey

Iron

Needed for healthy red blood cells (hemoglobin production), energy, good mood, attention, high IQ, and proper immune function

Found in: green leafy vegetables, kelp, beets, asparagus, carrots, cucumbers, watercress, parsley, grapes, bananas, figs, dried fruits, cherry juice, beans, soybeans, sunflower seeds, meats, fish, poultry, peas, eggs, whole grains, parsley, turmeric, seaweed, lentils, millet, pumpkin and sesame seeds, and blackstrap molasses

Potassium

Helps with maintenance of muscles and nerves and distributes and balances water in the body

Found in: spinach, celery, mushrooms, pecans, avocados, brussels sprouts, potatoes, legumes, all fruit, tomatoes, dried fruits, green vegetables, cantaloupe, pomegranates, whole grains, and sunflower seeds

Phosphorus

Needed for strong bones and teeth, cell growth and repair, energy production, healthy heart, hormone secretions, kidney function, nerve and muscle activity, and is used along with magnesium and calcium in acid/alkaline balance

Found in: squash, carrots, mushrooms, legumes, pumpkin and sesame seeds, whole grain cereals, oats, nuts, fish, meats, poultry, eggs, milk and milk products, and beans

Iodine

Needed for proper development of thyroid hormone, energy production, and physical and mental development

Found in: kelp, carrots, cod-liver oil, onions, seaweed, spinach, eggs, dairy, beets, celery, lettuce, mushrooms, grapes, oranges, seafood, and iodized salt

Selenium

Antioxidant, helps to prevent cancer, neutralizes heavy metals, slows the aging process, and works with vitamin E

Found in: whole grains, wheat germ, wheat bran, brewer's yeast, Brazil nuts, eggs, garlic, onions, salmon, barley, oats, brown rice, sunflower seeds, sesame seeds, swordfish, tuna, and herring

Zinc

Important for growth, skin repair, and carbohydrate digestion, and essential for the immune system, sexual development, and reproduction

Found in: mushrooms, asparagus, oats, wheat germ, brewer's yeast, soybeans, pumpkin and sunflower seeds, seafood, meats, organ meats, oysters, herring, eggs, dark meat poultry, miso, seaweed, buckwheat, ginger root, and black pepper

Essential Fatty Acids (EFAs)

Important for brain, nerve, and eye development, alertness, IQ, energy, skin condition, and heart function

OMEGA-3 (AND DHA): Helps memory loss, hyperactivity, and depression
Found in: tuna, herring, mackerel, sardines, salmon, cod-liver oil, walnuts, and flax seeds

OMEGA-6: Increases metabolism, energy and alleviates soft skin
Found in: flax seeds, almonds, Brazil nuts, hazelnuts, and sunflower, pumpkin, and sesame seeds and their oils

Protein

Important for growth and development, energy, healthy immune system, and hormonal balance

Found in: meat, fish, poultry, dairy products, soy products, pulses, beans, eggs, legumes, millet, amaranth, quinoa, nuts, and seeds

Carbohydrates

Needed for energy, fibre, vitamins, and minerals

Found in: grains and cereals (bread, pasta, oats, wheat, and rice), vegetables, fruits, beans, and pulses

Notes

1 R. Douglas Wilson, "Pre-conceptional Vitamin/Folic Acid Supplementation 2007: The Use of Folic Acid in Combination with a Multivitamin Supplement for the Prevention of Neural Tube Defects and Other Congenital Anomalies," Joint SOGC-Motherisk Clinical Practice Guideline No. 201, JOGC (December 2007).

2 P. De Wals, F. Tairou, M.I. Van Allen, et al. "Reduction in Neural-Tube Defects after Folic Acid Fortification in Canada," *New England Journal of Medicine* 357, 2 (2007):135–142.

3 Dr. Nigel Plummer, "The Developmental Origins of Modern Disease—Are We Programmed to Develop Disease in the Womb?" Seroyal Conference, Toronto, May 10, 2009.

4 Kirsi Laitinen, presentation to ECO 2009: The 17th European Congress on Obesity, Amsterdam, the Netherlands, May 7, 2009.

5 S. Rautava et al., "Probiotics during Pregnancy and Breast-Feeding Might Confer Immunomodulatory Protection against Atopic Disease in the Infant," *Journal of Allergy and Clinical Immunology,* 109 (2002):119–121.

6 Plummer, "The Developmental Origins of Modern Disease."

7 Canadian Organic Growers, "Consumers and Standards" (2009), www.cog.ca/index.php?page=consumers-and-standards.

8 Ontario Ministry of Agriculture, Food and Rural Affairs, Introduction to Organic Farming, Factsheet No. 06-103 (November 2006), www.omafra.gov.on.ca/english/crops/facts/06-103.htm.

9 E. Dehlink, E.Yen, A.M. Leichtner, E.J. Hait, and E. Fiebiger, "First Evidence of a Possible Association between Gastric Acid Suppression during Pregnancy and Childhood Asthma: A Population-Based Register Study," *Clinical and Experimental Allergy,* 39:246–253.

10 Plummer, "The Developmental Origins of Modern Disease."

11 Bruce W. Hollis and Carol L. Wagner, "Nutritional Vitamin D Status during Pregnancy: Reasons for Concern," *Canadian Medical Association Journal,* 174, 9 (April 25, 2006):1287–1290.

12 Cynthia Good Mojab, "Sunlight Deficiency: Helping Breastfeeding Mothers Find the Facts," *LEAVEN,* 39, 4 (August–September 2003):75–79.

[13] E. Hyppönen, E. Läärä, A. Reunanen, M.R. Järvelin, and S.M. Virtanen, "Intake of Vitamin D and Risk of Type 1 Diabetes: A Birth-Cohort Study," *Lancet*, 3, 358(9292) (November 2001):1500–1503.

[14] M. Ala-Houhala, "25-Hydroxyvitamin D levels during Breast-feeding with or without Maternal or Infantile Supplementation of Vitamin D," *Journal of Pediatric Gastroenterology and Nutrition*, 4, 2 (1985):220–226.

[15] Public Health Agency of Canada, "Canadian Paediatric Surveillance Program—2003 Results" (November 8, 2004), www.phac-aspc.gc.ca/publicat/cpsp-pcsp03/page8-eng.php.

[16] Health Canada, "Nutrients of Special Concern for a Healthy Pregnancy: Iron" (April 3, 2008), www.hc-sc.gc.ca/fn-an/consultation/init/prenatal/iron-fer-cons-eng.php.

[17] S. Raj, M. Faridi, U. Rusia, and O. Singh, "A Prospective Study of Iron Status in Exclusively Breastfed Term Infants Up to 6 Months of Age," *International Breastfeeding Journal*, 1, 3 (March 2008):3.

[18] A. Prentice, "Calcium in Pregnancy and Lactation," *Annual Review of Nutrition*, 20 (2000):249–272.

[19] Carolee Bateson-Koch, *Allergies: Disease in Disguise* (Burnaby, BC: Alive Books, 1994).

[20] Dr. Shonna Masse, pediatric dentist, interview with the author, June 2009.

[21] Ibid.

[22] Dr. Robert Penning, pediatric dentist, interview with the author, June 8, 2009.

[23] Eleanor Bimla Schwarz, M. Roberta Ray, Alison M. Stuebe et al., "Duration of Lactation and Risk Factors for Maternal Cardiovascular Disease," *Obstetrics & Gynecology*, 113, 5 (May 2009):974–982.

[24] Lars A. Hanson, *Immunobiology of Human Milk: How Breastfeeding Protects Babies* (Amarillo, TX: Pharmasoft Publishing, 2004), 77.

[25] Ibid., 82.

[26] Ibid., 93.

[27] Clare E. Casey, Anne Smith, and Peifang Zhang, "Microminerals in Human and Animal Milks," in Robert G. Jensen (Ed.), *Handbook of Milk Composition* (San Diego: Academic Press, 1995):622–673.

[28] Rosine Bishara et al., "Nutrient Composition of Hindmilk Produced by Mothers of Very Low Birth Weight Infants Born at Less Than 28 Week's Gestation," *Journal of Human Lactation*, 24, 2 (2008):159–167.

[29] Mary Frances Picciano, "Vitamins in Milk," in Jensen, *Handbook of Milk Composition*, 675–687.

[30] Timo, Saarela, Jorma Kokkenen, and Maila Koivisto, "Macronutrient and Energy Contents of Human Milk Fractions during the First Six Months of Lactation," *Acta Paediatrica*, 94 (2005):1176–1181.

[31] Jan Riordan and Kathleen G. Auerbach, *Breastfeeding and Human Lactation* (Boston: Jones and Bartlett, 1993).

32 Margit Hamosh, "Enzymes in Human Milk," in Jensen, *Handbook of Milk Composition*, 388–427.

33 Bo Lonnerdal and Stephanie Atkinson, "Nitrogenous Components of Milk," in Jensen, *Handbook of Milk Composition*, 351–368.

34 Hanson, *Immunobiology of Human Milk*, 83.

35 Ibid., 91.

36 Ibid.

37 Ibid., 83.

38 Ibid., 97.

39 S.S. Yalçin, A. Baykan, K. Yurdakök, S. Yalçin, and A.I. Gücüfl, "The Factors That Affect Milk-to-Serum Ratio for Iron during Early Lactation," *Journal of Pediatric Hematology/Oncology*, 31, 2 (February 2009): 85–90.

40 Riordan and Auerbach, *Breastfeeding and Human Lactation*.

41 Dr. Nigel Plummer, "Choosing the Right Probiotics for Your Patient," Seroyal Teleconference, Toronto, May 6, 2009.

42 Plummer, "The Developmental Origins of Modern Disease."

43 Riordan and Auerbach, *Breastfeeding and Human Lactation*.

44 Natalie Rogers, child birth educator, email interview with the author, June 8, 2009.

45 Ibid.

46 Jack Newman, *Dr. Jack Newman's Guide to Breastfeeding* (Toronto: HarperCollins, 2000), 80.

47 "Infant Formula: The Canadian Study" (July 3, 2004), www.truthinlabeling.org/formulacopy.html.

48 Online survey of 216 moms sent out by sproutright.com, facebook/canadianbabies.ca, weewelcome.ca, and meetup.com, June 8, 2009.

49 Beate Lloyd, Robin J. Halter, Mathew J. Kuchan et al., "Formula Tolerance in Postbreastfed and Exclusively Formula-Fed Infants," *Pediatrics*, 103, 1 (January 1999):e7.

50 W.W.K. Koo et al., "Reduced Bone Mineralization in Infants Fed Palm Olein-Containing Formula: A Randomized, Double-Blinded, Prospective Trial," *Pediatrics*, 111 (2003):1017–1023.

51 Charlotte Vallaeys, *DHA/ARA: Replacing Mother—Imitating Human Breast Milk in the Laboratory* (Cornucopia, WI: Cornucopia Institute, January 2008).

52 K. Kennedy et al., "Double-Blinded, Randomized Trial of a Synthetic Triacylglycerol in Formula-Fed Term Infants: Effects on Stool Biochemistry, Stool Characteristics, and Bone Mineralization," *American Journal of Clinical Nutrition*, 70 (1999):920–927.

53 Catherine L. Witt (September 15, 2006), www.medscape.com/viewarticle/544436.

54 Jeffrey M. Smith, *Genetic Roulette: The Documented Health Risks of Genetically Engineered Foods* (Fairfield, IA: Yes! Books, 2007).

55 Ibid.

[56] J.B. Lasekan, K.M. Ostrom, J.R. Jacobs et al., "Growth of Newborn, Term Infants Fed Soy Formulas for One Year," *Clinical Pediatrics*, 38 (1999):563–571.

[57] "NANNYcare Goat Milk Nutrition," NANNYcare home page (2007), www.vitacare.co.uk/ProductInfo.aspx.

[58] "Types of Lactose Intolerance," foodreactions.org (2005), www.foodreactions.org/intolerance/lactose/types.html.

[59] Julia Moskin, "For an All-Organic Formula, Baby, That's Sweet," *New York Times* (May 19, 2008), www.nytimes.com/2008/05/19/us/19formula.html?_r=1.

[60] K. Kennedy et al., "Double-Blinded, Randomized Trial."

[61] Ibid.

[62] Online survey sent out by sproutright.com, facebook/canadianbabies.ca, weewelcome.ca, and meetup.com, June 8, 2009.

[63] Ontario Association of Osteopathic Manual Practitioners home page (December 17, 2009), www.osteopathyontario.com.

[64] Tema Stein, pediatric osteopath, interview with the author, June 8, 2009.

[65] I. Alexandrovich , O. Rakovitskaya, E. Kolmo, T. Sidorova, and I. Shushunov, "The Effect of Fennel (Foeniculum Vulgare) Seed Oil Emulsion in Infantile Colic: A Randomized, Placebo-Controlled Study," *Alternative Therapies in Health and Medicine*, 4 (July/August 2003):58–61.

[66] Bastyr Center for Natural Health, "Herbal Combination Relieves Colic in Babies" (2009), http://bastyrcenter.org/content/view/943/&page=.

[67] Plummer, "Choosing the Right Probiotics."

[68] Health Canada, "Food Allergies and Intolerances" (June 5, 2009), www.hc-sc.gc.ca/fn-an/securit/allerg/index-eng.php.

[69] Susan F. Plummer, Iveta Garaiova, Tinnu Sarvotham et al., "Effects of Probiotics on the Composition of the Intestinal Microbiota Following Antibiotic Therapy," *International Journal of Antimicrobial Agents*, 26 (2005):69–74.

[70] "Our History: Alan Brown," The Hospital for Sick Children (SickKids), www.sickkids.ca/AboutSickKids/History-and-Milestones/Our-History/Alan-Brown.html.

[71] G.Y. Du Toit, P. Katz, P. Sasieni et al., "Early Consumption of Peanuts in Infancy Is Associated with a Low Prevalence of Peanut Allergy," *Journal of Allergy and Clinical Immunology*, 122, 5 (November 2008):984–991.

[72] L. Mondoulet, E. Paty, M.F. Drumare et al., "Influence of Thermal Processing on the Allergenicity of Peanut Proteins," *Journal of Agricultural and Food Chemistry*, 53 (2005):4547–4553.

[73] F. Sanchez-Valverde, F. Gil, D. Martinez et al., "The Impact of Caesarean Delivery and Type of Feeding on Cow's Milk Allergy in Infants and Subsequent Development of Allergic March in Childhood," *Allergy*, 64, 6 (June 2009):884–889.

[74] Bateson-Koch, Allergies, 54.

[75] Bateson-Koch, Allergies.

76 Janet Neilson, homeopath, interview with the author, June 8, 2009.

77 "About Organic Produce," www.ocf.berkeley.edu/~lhom/organictext.html.

78 www.whatsonmyfood.org.

79 Riordan and Auerbach, *Breastfeeding and Human Lactation*.

80 Online survey sent out via sproutright.com, weewelcome.ca, facebook/
canadianbabies.ca, and meetup.com, June 8, 2009.

81 Interview with Tracey Ruiz, "The Sleep Doula," June 8, 2009.

82 Online survey sent out via sproutright.com, weewelcome.ca, facebook/
canadianbabies.ca, and meetup.com, June 8, 2009.

83 Ibid.

84 George A. Wootan, "Breast Feeding: New Discoveries," The Natural Child Project,
www.naturalchild.org/guest/george_wootan.html.

85 The Food Allergy and Anaphylaxis Network, "Allergens: Tree Nuts," http://www.
foodallergy.org/page/tree-nuts1.

86 Valerie Elliot, "Cow&Gate and Farley's Rusks Attacked for Fat, Sugar and Salt
Content," *The Times* (May 5, 2009),
www.timesonline.co.uk/tol/news/uk/health/article6216207.ece.

87 "Baby Mum-Mum (Original): Product Info" (2009), www.mummums.com/
products/baby-mum-mums.

88 "Family Nutrition," AskDr.Sears.com (2006), www.askdrsears.com/html/4/
t041100.asp.

89 Siegfried Gursche, *Good Fats and Oils, Alive Natural Health Guide 17* (Burnaby,
BC: Alive Books, 2009).

90 Dr. Richard Mass, interview on *Marketplace*, CBC (March 2001), www.cbc.ca/
consumers/market/files/health/leadwater/index.html.

ACKNOWLEDGMENTS

Thank you, thank you, thank you. So many people were involved in helping writing this book.

Firstly, thank you to every mom and dad I meet in my workshops, Mommy Chef cooking classes, and trade shows, and speak with on the phone. You're why I do what I do, and I feel honoured to support you through such an important time in your lives. Beth, whom I could not have written this book without—thank you for running my company while I wrote for months, as well as for staying up late with me when needed! To my personal editor and sister, Janine, who helped me beyond words. To my research team of nutrition students, who searched for the most current information they could find: Elizabeth, Marta, Marlene, Betty, Meredith, and Natalie. To Julia from the Institute of Holistic Nutrition for finding me such a great team. And to my fellow mom-entrepreneurs, who supported me by sending out my survey to their followers and helped me keep it together.

Thank you to all the experts who allowed me to pick their clever brains and gain insight into their areas of expertise: dentists Dr. Dana Colson, Dr. Shonna Masse, and Dr. Robert Penning; osteopath Tema Stein; The Sleep Doula, Tracey Ruiz; homeopath Janet Neilson; and child birth educator Natalie Rogers.

To the great editorial team at Penguin Canada for the opportunity to write this book: Andrea Magyar, acquisitions editor; Helen Smith, associate editor; David Ross, production editor; and Marcia Gallego, copy editor. The stars must have been aligned one morning in January 2009 when I called into CHUM FM as a listener (responding to a question about probiotics). Andrea heard me on the radio and got in touch, and that was the beginning of this fantastic venture!

Thank you to my role model—my mum. Healthy eating and cooking seasonal foods from scratch was our way of life growing up. Although I didn't like eating granola while my friends ate chips and chocolate at school, it gave me a lifelong understanding of healthy eating, and I'm healthier for it. It has inspired me to cook for my girls in the same way.

And last, but certainly not least, to my husband, Chris, and daughters, Logan, and Hadley, for giving me the time to write this book. I know it was hard to understand why Mommy couldn't play or go to Gramma and Grampa's with you on the weekends. Thank you for your love, patience, and support (hugs and kisses, too!).

INDEX